The
PIZZA
DIET

The PIZZA DIET

How I Lost 100 Pounds Eating My Favorite Food— and You Can Too!

Pasquale Cozzolino

And the Editors of *Eat This, Not That!*

To everyone who wants to live a leaner, healthier life while still enjoying food to the fullest. May this book provide a delicious way to manage your hunger and become a more mindful eater.

No book can replace the diagnostic expertise and medical advice of a trusted physician. Please be certain to consult with your doctor before making any decisions that affect your health, particularly if you suffer from any medical condition or have any symptom that may require treatment.

Mention of specific companies, organizations, or authorities in this book does not imply endorsement by the author or publisher, nor does mention of specific companies, organizations, or authorities imply that they endorse this book, its author, or the publisher.

Published in the United States by Galvanized Books, a division of Galvanized Brands, LLC, New York

Galvanized Books is a trademark of Galvanized Brands, LLC

ISBN 978-0-399-17996-9

Printed in the United States of America on acid-free paper

Interior design by Judy Ross

Interior photography by Jennifer May

Cover design by Joseph Heroun

Cover photograph by Getty

GALVANIZED

CONTENTS

My Lifesaving Recipe

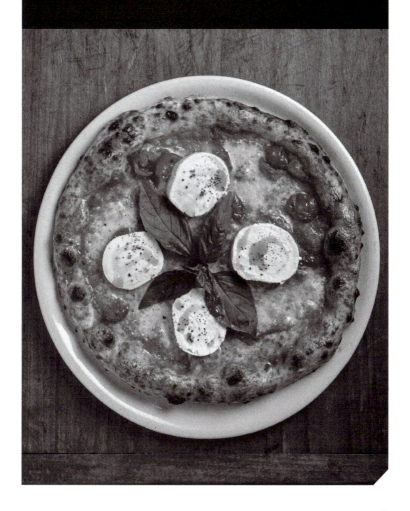

I WOKE UP ONE DAY AND I NOTICED I COULDN'T SEE MY FEET.

MY STOMACH WAS IN THE WAY.

It was August 2015. I tipped the scale at an enormous 370 pounds. My doctor told me to stop eating so much. "If you keep this up," she warned me, "you'll be dead of a heart attack soon."

It wasn't always this way. When I came to New York from Naples in 2011, I weighed 254 pounds, which is fairly healthy for a guy who stands 6-foot-6. I had a dream of opening my own restaurant, but I needed investors, and investors had to be convinced I could run it myself. So I did my research. I rushed around New York City tasting every new experience, visiting two or three restaurants a day. One day, I'd visit a restaurant posing as a reporter from Italy and ask all the questions I could think of. The next, I'd just eat my way through the menu. When you eat and eat, your stomach stretches, and mine did. To feel satisfied, you have to eat more. I ate a *lot* more.

It began with an occasional soda. And then something tasty and fast to go with it. Fast food made me feel good—for a moment. When you're trying to build a career and raise a family, you're hustling; everything else isn't so important—like what you're eating. You grab whatever's easy and fast. It never occurred to me, but I'd stopped paying attention to food, and I ignored what poor eating was doing to my body. I just bought bigger pants. Here I was an expert in food, a chef who had spent years studying how to create healthy meals with the freshest ingredients, and I was eating myself to death with junk food.

My wife Jordie and friends noticed the change in me, and they started to get upset. "Okay," I said, "I'll take care of it." But I didn't. And then I couldn't bend over to pick up my son at the playground. There was a hundred pounds of fat between me and my Francesco.

I had dangerously high cholesterol, shockingly low good cholesterol, with triglycerides at 464 when they should've been under 150. My doctor pleaded with me, "Think about your wife, your young son, and the second child on the way."

That woke me up. I finally realized I had a responsibility to survive. And if I wanted to survive, I had to change.

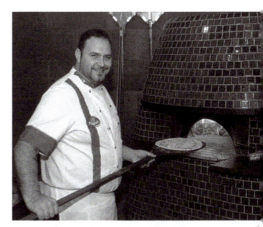

EXTRA CHEESE: At my heaviest, I weighed 370 pounds. It was time to get serious about my diet.

I had tried diets before, of course, but I found that I could never stick to them. I would drop a few pounds, then lose the discipline to continue and ultimately gain all the weight back. You've heard the statistics: Between 80 and 95 percent of people who diet end up putting weight back on and then some. Is it the dieter who fails, or is the diet so restrictive that it's too difficult to follow? At the doctor's office, in that moment, I resolved that whatever changes I made this time had to be permanent. I would find a way to lose weight on my terms and keep it off for good. But I needed a strategy that was different from my previous attempts to lose weight.

That summer I went home to Naples and ran into an old friend who'd lost a lot of weight. I asked him how he did it. He introduced me to Giovanni Moscarella, an Italian nutritionist who's famous for his book *Dieta Biosofica* (Bio-Philosophy of Diet). Giovanni told me, "Pasquale, a diet you don't like, you're never going to follow. You have to eat something that tastes good to you."

I realized Giovanni had given me something of a riddle. He wasn't going to solve my problem for me. He knew I couldn't just go out and radically change the way I ate overnight. I couldn't, like magic, change my lifestyle and expect to stick with it. I was so hooked on bad food habits that no eating plan I tried felt right. How could I find something that I really wanted to eat but wasn't fattening?

A SLICE OF LIFE

The neighborhood where I grew up, Quartieri Spagnoli, was the poorest in Naples. Our family had just enough money to get by. My mother was a housewife, and my father sold electrical supplies. We lived in a tiny apartment where I shared a bedroom with my two sisters. There was never extra money for luxuries, but every Saturday night my parents would take us out to try a different pizzeria. In the historic center of Naples, there are over 600 pizzerias; there were choices everywhere. On Saturdays as dinnertime approached, I'd jump around the house with excitement. Neapolitan families got together over pizza; there was no food in the Quartieri I loved more. When I say to my son now, we're going for pizza, he jumps up just like I used to. Pizza has that childlike power. It's a special food, with a mix of flavors and textures that complement each other perfectly. It is no wonder that so many people around the world say it's their favorite food. The first time I ate pizza, I couldn't have been more than 2 years old. My parents recalled that it was love at first bite.

Pizza was invented in Naples, and it's always going to be the basis for Neapolitan food. Growing up there, I always wanted more pizza. More and more and more. As a boy, I'd already made a decision: "One day I will be a pizza maker so I can eat pizza every day."

My parents, unfortunately, had different ideas. When I turned 13, I was desperate to enroll in the local culinary high school on top of Posillipo Hill overlooking the entire Gulf of Naples. IPSSAR Ippolito Cavalcanti was one of the biggest cooking schools in all of Italy. The school had everything I wanted. Students got 30 hours a week of food training. Classes were taught by famous Italian chefs. If you wanted to be a chef in Italy, this was the school to attend.

But my parents had other plans for me. They said no to culinary school; they signed me up for the economics school. Working in a kitchen was no life for their son, they said. It was hot, sweaty work with long hours and low pay.

So I went to economics school. And I hated it. After a year there, I sat my parents down and pleaded with them to let me change schools. The next fall, I was on my way.

From my first day, it was thrilling. My teacher said he wasn't going to mislead us: "This is a tough life. We work hard when everybody else is having fun." I didn't care. Let's go forward, I said.

In the next 5 years, I learned almost everything there was to know about Italian and French cuisine. How to turn potatoes into gnocchi, how to bake delicious dessert and, of course, how to create the classic Neapolitan pizza. After graduating, I landed a job in the food-service world working alongside my cousin Maurizio Gambino as a caterer backstage at rock concerts. The company, called Giromangiando, cooked for some of the world's biggest acts—U2, Muse and Coldplay—and while it may sound glamorous, it was as tough a life as my teacher had said it would be on that first day of school.

It was a crazy life. I was tired after 10 years on the road, traveling from city to city in the back of a cramped tour bus. I wanted to put down roots and have a family, but there was no opportunity in Naples. And that's when I got an offer to come to America. It was my chance to be a pizza chef for a restaurant. It was my dream come true. But during those first few stressful years in the United States, the lifestyle change transformed my body. I put on more than 100 pounds eating American fast food—burgers, fries, cola, and often as many as six pizzas a day! When you're skinny for your whole life and you suddenly get fat, your body isn't used to carrying so much weight and it starts to break down. The weight took its toll on my entire body. I felt horrible. I had back pain, knee pain, acid reflux, chest pain, terrible migraines, and anxiety.

Giovanni's riddle continued to haunt me. The nutritionist told me, for any diet to work, I had to find something I loved to eat that would satisfy my cravings but wouldn't make me fatter. I had to learn to eat fewer calories, which is very difficult to do, especially for a chef whose work and life are surrounded by amazing food! But how?

MY *DOUGH!* MOMENT

Back in Naples, as I walked through Quartieri Spagnoli one evening, it hit me—the smoky scent of cooking pizza brought back wonderful childhood memories. That was it! Pizza! Pizza, the most important food in my life. Pizza, the reason I became a chef. If I cannot have pizza, I reasoned, I cannot follow a diet. But what if I could make a healthier style? Knowing there's a pizza waiting for me in the middle of each day, I could follow any diet. That gave me the motivation to push forward and develop my Pizza Diet.

I experimented with ways to make pizza healthier and lower in calories. I started with the techniques from back home in Naples and put my own spin on them. My pizza would be made with high-quality ingredients, and the dough would be the secret ingredient.

Most pizzas in the United States are made with highly-processed white flour, which is very inexpensive. The downside is that this white flour pizza isn't very healthy for you. It is really no better than white sandwich bread, and it raises your blood sugar just as rapidly.

For my pizza, I use a stone-milled flour that's more nutritious because the grain is ground between two heavy stones; it's less-processed and contains some of the germ and bran. The dough makes the pizza crust lighter and more flavorful. This special flour needs to be fermented for a long time so the yeast can make the dough rise and the gluten can be adequately broken down. It is certainly a more-expensive and time-consuming process, but it is worth the effort because the result will help you lose weight deliciously.

My special dough recipes, shared in this book for the first time, will help you become leaner and healthier.

▶ **You'll reduce cravings and stay fuller longer.** Studies have shown that the larger particle size in stone-ground flour compared to industrially-milled flour reduces its Glycemic Index, meaning it's slower to absorb into the bloodstream and will cause less of a spike in your blood sugar. By slowing carbohydrate breakdown into sugar, you stay full longer and avoid blood sugar spikes and dips that can trigger overeating.

▶ **You'll lose weight quickly.** When I knew that I could enjoy my favorite food—pizza—every day, I felt a weight lifted off my shoulders. I did not get anxious about denying myself food, and I found that it was much easier to control calories and portion sizes throughout the day. Within the first week, the pounds started to melt away.

▶ **You'll virtually eliminate gluten sensitivity.** I have gluten-free friends who cannot eat any other pizza but mine. That's because the 36-hour fermentation process during which my Pizza Diet dough rises breaks down most of the bread's gluten.

▶ **You'll live your healthiest, happiest life!** In addition to eating my weight-loss pizza for lunch, you'll enjoy a healthy breakfast and light dinner based on the Mediterranean Diet. That's the typical way of eating in countries bordering the Mediterranean Sea, which focuses on fresh vegetables, fruits, fish, whole grains, and healthy fats like olive oil and avocado. It's the way

I used to eat when I lived in Italy, and I'd replaced it with fast food and sugary processed foods when I came to New York City. The Mediterranean Diet is associated with lowering bad cholesterol and reducing risk of heart disease and cancer.

Along with my beloved pizza, following the Mediterranean Diet became my savior. In the first 2 weeks on the Pizza Diet, I lost 20 pounds. When you see that kind of progress, it gives you motivation. It gives you confidence in your conviction and makes you want to do more. I even signed up for a kickboxing class at my local gym. My weight kept dropping at about 3 pounds per week, and I quickly began to feel better. My mood changed. I was happier. Even sexually, things improved, but enough said about that! People told me I looked younger. I had more energy. I could run and climb stairs without becoming winded.

Best of all, I started to love myself again. My confidence returned. The most beautiful feeling was when I pulled out from the back of the closet a pair of old jeans, and I could actually fit into them again. When I had first started my diet, my wife told me to throw away all my old clothes because I'd never wear them again. I realize now that was just her sneaky way of motivating me to lose weight. I am so grateful to her for pushing and supporting me to take action.

In the first 9 months of the Pizza Diet, I shed 114 pounds and completely turned my life around. I no longer craved junk food. It's amazing; once you start eating fresh, healthy foods, your body rejects the crap. It begins to tell you how you should be eating. You get into a rhythm. Even portion control becomes easier.

I understand how it is for people with extra pounds. They

feel so frustrated, so hopeless. They feel terrible because they can't do everything they might like. Even worse, their weight affects their self-esteem. I was that way, too. It's emotionally discouraging and exhausting. And I never want to go back to that place.

When people see me now, they ask how I lost so much weight and how I did it. When I tell them about the Pizza Diet, I can tell they are a little skeptical. "Are you sure?" they'll ask with a puzzled look on their faces.

I'm sure.

My weight-loss story has gone around the globe. I was on the front page of the *New York Post* and featured in magazines and newspapers in South America, Asia, Australia, Europe, and Russia. People are fascinated by my example. They are amazed and encouraged when they see my before-and-after pictures. It proves to them that if I can do it, they can do it. I am living proof that you really can heal your body with food. And you can do it with delicious pizza—no joke. This book will show you how.

Chapter 1

The Pizza Diet Secret

The simple principles for weight-loss success

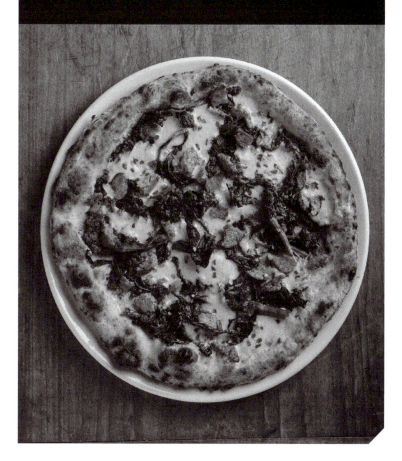

I know what you're thinking, because I had my doubts, too. The idea of a pizza diet sounds ridiculous at first—like an oxymoron—or worse yet, like just another in the endless parade of weight-loss gimmicks we've been subjected to for decades, from the cookie diet, to the grapefruit diet to something called the "werewolf" diet, where meals are based on the lunar calendar.

But this is no fad, and I have my medical paperwork and the before-and-after photos to prove it to you. I lost more than 100 pounds in 9 months and reversed several health problems that stemmed from weighing far more than I should have.

How is it possible to eat pizza every day and still lose weight, you ask? It starts with redefining how we think of pizza. Made correctly, pizza is filled with a mix of nutrients that make it a truly nutritious meal. It's only fattening junk food if it's made quickly and cheaply with low-quality ingredients the way most pizza is dished out in the United States. Most dough used by American pizzerias is nutritionally deficient and loaded with preservatives and hydrogenated fat. The cheese is greasy, and the toppings are often frozen. If that's the kind of pizza you're eating, your body is going to suffer.

My pizza is different. It's made in the old Italian way, with fresh produce and special dough, and it fits nicely into a diverse, well-rounded diet.

Despite what's been drummed into our heads over the last few years, not all carbs are bad. They make up an important part of our diet, and they're essential for our body to function properly. They provide energy, reduce the risk of cardiovascular disease, and the fiber contained in many types (including fruits, vegetables and whole grains) helps us feel fuller and keeps our weight down. (Studies have also shown that eating foods with our hands, such as pizza, helps us feel more satisfied because it helps us experience greater aroma and texture of our food.)

The plan I lay out in this book is based on the Mediterranean Diet, that way of eating based on the old traditions of Greece and southern Italy, where the rates of chronic disease are among the lowest in the world and the life expectancy is highest. This is what I grew up with; this is the food I love.

The Mediterranean Diet is often represented as a pyramid, with the food groups you should eat most appearing at the bottom and those you should steer clear of at the top. The majority of our calories should come from plant sources: fruits, vegetables, potatoes, seeds, nuts and yes, whole grains, including flour and bread. Next is seafood and healthy oils, such as the only one I generally use in my kitchen: extra-virgin olive oil. Then you have poultry, eggs, and dairy, which should be consumed in relatively small amounts, and finally at the top of the pyramid, you have red meat and desserts. Try to eat those only a few times a month.

While some things like meat and sweets should be consumed in moderation, I don't believe in trying to completely excise certain food groups from your diet. Our cells are regenerating every day, and our bodies need to have available every component from food—carbs, protein, sugar, fat, vitamins, minerals, cholesterol, everything. We need all of these things, but only in the right amounts.

The Mediterranean Diet mandates getting about half of your calories from carbohydrates, 20 percent from protein and 30 percent from fat, and that's roughly the parameters of my Pizza Diet plan. Here's what it looks like right out of the oven:

THE PIZZA DIET AT A GLANCE

Lose weight and belly fat without sacrificing your favorite foods! You'll enjoy three meals and snacks, including pizza!

WHAT TO EAT:

▶ **Mediterranean Diet foods,** such as fresh vegetables, fruits, whole grains, seafood, and lean proteins. (See the expanded list on 55.)

▶ **One personal pizza for lunch** made with my special Pizza Diet dough.

▶ **One or two snacks** to take the edge off hunger when needed. Focus on proteins, fruits, and vegetables.

WHAT TO DRINK:

▶ **Zero-calorie beverages** every day (mostly water and unsweetened iced tea), and a glass of red wine on occasion.

WHEN TO EAT:

▶ **Start with breakfast** before 9 a.m., lunch at 1, and a light dinner no later than 7 p.m. Eat one or two snacks in between meals.

CHEAT DAY:

▶ **One day a week,** eat whatever you like, but don't go crazy. A cheat day isn't for your stomach. It's for your mind.

WHAT TO LIMIT:

▶ **Red meat,** especially highly processed meats like salami.

▶ **Ice cream and desserts.** Sweets pack on pounds, cause inflammation, and contribute to insulin resistance that can lead to diabetes. Limit yourself to 5 teaspoons of added sugars per day.

▶ **Processed carbohydrates.** Snacking on chips, crackers, and baked goods only fans the flames of cravings. Avoid these empty-calorie foods.

▶ **Alcohol.** Research suggest that an occasional glass of red wine may offer health benefits. But if you take alcohol out of the picture, you'll lose weight faster. Alcohol encourages fat storage.

WHEN TO EXERCISE:

▶ **Daily,** if possible. At least five times a week, get 30 to 60 minutes of moderately intense exercise. Start with walking, if you're out of shape, and increase intensity over time with more rigorous activity like running, swimming, cycling, or strength training.

WHEN TO STOP:

▶ **Depending on your starting weight,** it can take 4 weeks or more (for me, 9 months) to reach your goal weight. You can stop eating one pizza a day, if you wish, after you have lost more than 10 pounds and established healthy eating habits.

PIZZA DIET DETAILS—
WHAT YOU'LL DO:

EAT FOUR OR FIVE TIMES A DAY

Our bodies need to be fed frequently so we keep our metabolism revving and we don't switch to fat-storage mode. I recommend eating three modest meals a day, with healthy snacks (usually fruit and protein) in between. I have breakfast around 8 a.m., lunch at 1 p.m., and dinner no later than 6 p.m. Then I eat nothing else for the rest of the night. You can have meals at different times, say breakfast at 10, or maybe dinner at 5 or 7 p.m. But try not to each much later than 7 p.m. A full stomach may make it difficult to get to sleep. If you don't sleep well, you pack on the pounds.

Studies show that people who are sleep deprived and fatigued tend to crave carbohydrates the next day. In fact, researchers say that people who get fewer than 6 hours of sleep per night end up eating close to 300 more calories per day than people who get 7 to 8 hours of sleep a night. Give yourself time to burn off some calories before bedtime, and ensure a good night's rest.

EAT LIKE THEY DO IN SICILY

Fill up on whole grains, seafood and lean proteins. And, of course, pizza. I have one pizza every day for lunch, changing up the toppings to keep my taste buds interested. Breakfast typically consists of whole-grain cereal (remember, I cook for a living, so I try to avoid spending a lot of time in the kitchen when I'm home). And I keep dinners light—often just a protein, simply grilled, with a side of vegetables. Easy. Uncomplicated by heavy sauces and starches.

No matter what you eat, you usually can't go wrong if you eat naturally and choose the best ingredients you possibly can—fresh fruits and vegetables, organic when possible. Enjoy them when they're in season.

NEVER SACRIFICE

Stick to this plan 6 days a week, then on the seventh, allow yourself a cheat day, during which you can eat whatever you like. I'm not going to put limits on your cheat day, but be realistic. You're trying to lose weight here. I wouldn't go too crazy. The purpose of the cheat day isn't about your stomach anyway. It's about your mind.

When I first started the Pizza Diet, I found the luxury of a cheat day was vital to keeping me sane. Sure, I had my pizza. But early on, the prospect of never eating another french fry or bowl of ice cream virtually left me sobbing into my penne. I needed a cheat day for the emotional benefit of knowing I could still indulge on occasion. As I began to eat healthier, however, I found that the cheat day became less and less important to me. By about 3 months into the Pizza Diet, I no longer craved junk food at all. The sodium was too much. The taste of greasy food began to disgust me. I would sit down on my cheat day to a slice of cake, take one bite, then push the plate away. Too sweet. Gross. No, thank you.

See how you feel as you progress on the Pizza Diet. You may get to a place where you can skip the cheat day altogether. Wouldn't that feel amazing?

EAT MINDFULLY

This healthy way of eating in moderation is not about constantly saying *no, no, no* to your favorite foods. After all, you can have pizza! You can have a cheat day, if you wish. But a critical element of Pizza Diet success is becoming much more mindful of what you are putting in your mouth the rest of the time. Limiting or eliminating certain not-so-good-for-you foods will improve your health and accelerate your weight loss.

For example, you should try to reduce your consumption of red meat. Sure, it's a great source of protein, but red meat also contains high amounts of saturated fat, sodium, nitrites, and carcinogens that occur during high-heat cooking. Processed red meat should be first on your list to limit. In a study analyzing nearly 30 years of data on more than 120,000 adults, Harvard School of Public Health researchers linked daily consumption of processed meats, like salami, to a 20 percent increased risk of death. So if you like pepperoni on your pizza, save that topping for rare special occasions. And work toward replacing red meat with healthier sources of protein, such as fish, chicken, turkey, eggs, nuts, legumes, and dairy products.

Start skipping nightly ice cream and other desserts. Limit yourself to just 5 teaspoons of added sugar a day. Try to avoid foods made with GMOs (genetically modified organisms). The jury is still out on whether they're harmful or not. One day, studies might confirm that GMOs are safe to eat, but until then, I avoid them.

Also work toward removing all the junk food from your life, especially chips, crackers and candies, which deliver little nutrition and a lot of empty calories. I also avoid any of the food additives that are banned in Europe but still, for some reason, are legal here in the United States. Steer clear of unnatural preservatives, artificial colors and chemicals such as potassium bromate and azodicarbonamide (both used in baked goods), rBGH (a hormone given to dairy cows) and brominated vegetable oil (a chemical used in soft drinks that contains the element bromine, which is used in flame retardants).

HOW I LOST 100 POUNDS

I completely cut out the liquid calories. They go down too easy and you don't realize you're getting them. I was drinking three cans of soda a day. When I stopped, I felt the difference.

TOP IT WITH EXERCISE

You'll lose more weight if you do. The combination of a healthy Mediterranean-style diet and regular exercise is powerful for weight loss and maintenance. What's more, exercise is one of the best things you can do to reduce your risk of disease. A report published in the *Journal of the American Medical Association*, for example, found that those who coupled exercise with the Mediterranean Diet decreased their chance of getting Alzheimer's by an astounding 60 percent.

Exercise brings you many, many more health benefits. It improves your mood and your ability to think clearly. Scientific research has shown that exercise can be in some cases as effective as anti-depressant medication at relieving symptoms of clinical depression. Exercise boosts your brainpower and it strengthens the immune system helping to fend off germs and illnesses. Exercise keeps your arteries flexible. Consider learning how to lift some weights if you haven't tried. Building some muscle through resistances training burns calories when you are exercising and also afterward when your muscles use calories to repair and grow.

Whatever type of workout you choose—walking, running, biking, swimming, weight lifting or sport—try for 30 to 60 minutes of moderately intense exercise five times a week.

KEEP IT UP

How long do you stay on the Pizza Diet? Well, it's not a 4-week crash diet you use to get into shape for swimsuit season and then discard in the fall. This is a lifestyle, and as long as you follow the general principles I lay out here, you can continue eating like this as long as you like. You will lose significant pounds within the first two weeks and and may continue to drop more until you reach your goal weight. That doesn't mean you have to eat a pizza for lunch every day, forever or even until you hit your goal if you don't want to. Pizza at lunch just makes eating a light Mediterranean-style dinner easier. You can even swap out the pizza for a healthy pasta, a nice salad, or chicken sandwich, in the name of variety. The Pizza Diet is about establishing healthy eating habits while still enjoying your must-have food.

Chapter 2

Beat Your Carb Addiction

How to break free of sugar's grip

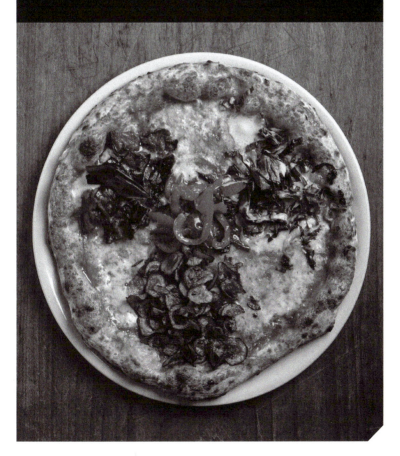

I read a statistic recently that the average American man weighed 166 pounds in the 1960s but now weighs about 190 pounds. The average woman in the '60s weighed 140; today she weighs 164.

The Centers for Disease Control says 70 percent of Americans over age 20 are either overweight or obese. How did Americans get so fat so fast? I have to believe it's the same way I ballooned to 370 pounds when I moved here from Italy. I ate too much. I consumed too many calories from fast food and processed foods with added sugars. In America, portion sizes are enormous. When I learned to bake muffins in culinary school, muffins were about 2 ounces. Today, New York deli muffins weigh 8 ounces and contain as much as 400 calories. I've eaten my share of them. When I was starting out here I was under a lot of stress, so I craved carbohydrates. I wasn't eating the fresh produce that was a staple of my diet back in Italy. I drank a lot of soda, and you've seen how large fountain sodas have become. A large isn't 8 ounces anymore; it's 32 ounces, and then you can even supersize it!

Much has been written about America's carbohydrate addiction, and I've experienced it, as you can see from my "before-the-Pizza-Diet" photo on 11. Carbs made me dangerously overweight.

What is it about carbs that's so addictive? To answer that, it helps to first understand what we are talking about when we say "carbohydrates." Carbohydrate (sugar, really) is our body's main source of energy. We need it to survive. We get it by eating foods that contain carbs, like fruits, vegetables, grains, legumes, and sweeteners.

Not all carbs, however, are equal. There are *simple* carbs, which can be unhealthy, and *complex* carbs, which are more beneficial. Simple carbs, like those in fruit, soda, sugar and white breads, have one or two sugar molecules. As a result they digest and turn into energy superfast. That's fine if your muscles need a quick burst of energy. But the downside is that fast-digesting carbs also spike your blood sugar. If you eat a lot of simple carbs, that means your blood sugar spikes repetitively. Over time, frequent blood sugar spikes can trigger insulin resistance and, ultimately, diabetes.

Complex carbs, on the other hand, digest slowly, releasing a controlled, steady stream of energy into the bloodstream so they cause no wild blood sugar spikes. We get complex carbs from vegetables, legumes, whole grains like brown rice and quinoa, and whole-grain breads. What's the difference between white bread and whole-grain bread? Refining the flour to make white bread removes the slow-digesting fiber, turning it into a simple carb.

The reason you may love cupcakes, white bread, white rice, white pasta, chips, pretzels and, yes, most pizza has more to do with your brain than your stomach. Simple carbohydrates that digest quickly can stimulate the reward region of the brain—called the *nucleus accumbens*—involved in emotions, cravings and addiction, according to a study in the *American Journal of Clinical Nutrition*. Scientists monitoring brain scans of subjects who ate sugary foods actually saw those reward/addiction regions light up with activity.

Interestingly, eating proteins and fats, which digest slowly like complex carbs do, doesn't trigger those reward areas of the brain, which is why cravings for, say, steak or avocados are rare, unlike those for ice cream or chocolate cake.

One thing that scientists have found that makes carb cravings even worse is fatigue. Hormones that play a role in appetite and satiety are greatly influenced by lack of sleep. When you are tired from inadequate sleep, your brain craves carbohydrates for energy. Being tired also increases your mental stress, which causes your body to release the stress hormone cortisol, which also triggers hunger and cravings for carbs.

The solution to carb addiction, what helped me overcome it, is replacing highly processed simple carbohydrates with vegetables, whole grains, healthy fats and lean proteins, and finding a way to make my beloved pizza a healthy indulgence instead of yet another processed simple carb. I will explain how the Mediterranean way of eating helped me do that later in this book. But here are some other strategies to help you break free of carbohydrate addiction.

Rock steady. Keep your blood sugar levels level by eating at regular times every day (no skipping meals). And make sure you select lean proteins, healthy fats and complex carbs (vegetables and whole grains) over processed foods and simple carbs.

Cut out baked goods. Cookies, cakes, pastries. Get them out of your pantry. They only fuel cravings and blood sugar spikes. You'll get your baked-bread fix from a healthy pizza soon enough.

Eat more fiber. Most Americans get only about half the 20 to 30 grams of daily fiber they should. That means they are missing out on the best way to reduce cravings and fight diabetes. Because fiber isn't broken down in digestion, it doesn't raise blood sugar and actually slows down the flow of sugar into the bloodstream. Get your fiber from whole-grain cereals like oatmeal, low-sugar fruits like berries, apples, and grapefruit and vegetables, such as broccoli, kale, string beans, cauliflower, onions, peppers, beets, potatoes, and more. One study showed that people who ate 26 grams of fiber per day experienced an 18 percent reduction in their diabetes risk when compared to people who ate less than 19 grams a day.

HOW I LOST 100 POUNDS

I figured that if I can cut calories and still eat the Neapolitan pizza I love, I could lose weight on my terms.

Drink more water. Filling up on water (0 calories, remember) can keep you from overeating. Often people mistake thirst for hunger and reach for a fork instead of a glass of ice water. A study in the journal *Obesity* found that simply drinking a glass of water before meals helped people lose weight over a 12-week period. Unsweetened iced tea works, too. But stay away from diet soda. Studies show that people who drink diet soda have higher waist measurements and increased belly fat.

Go for grapefruit. Studies published in the *Journal of Medicinal Food* have found that citrus fruits like grapefruit, orange, and lemon have a positive effect on weight loss.

Avoid hidden sugars. Refined sugars are everywhere and in many surprising places, from yogurt, cereal and peanut butter to condiments and frozen pizza. The only way to avoid them is to become a food detective. Check labels and plan to be amazed.

Stop eating ultra-processed foods. Ultra-processed foods are the "formulation" of multiple processed ingredients. On top of the added salts and sugars, this "ultra" distinction includes substances not generally used in cooking like flavors, colors, emulsifiers, and other additives designed to imitate the qualities of "real food." So, what are these exactly? Think sodas, cheesy chips, chicken nuggets, and instant soups. According to a new study published in *BMJ Open*, additive-laden foods make up almost 60 percent of our daily calories. While ultra-processed foods are tailored to appeal to our taste buds, they're often lacking in valuable nutrients—like fiber, antioxidants, vitamins, and minerals—which have been found to combat and protect against the very same health issues that ultra-processed foods cause.

Don't let lettuce fool you. Just because there's lettuce and maybe a broccoli floret on your plate doesn't mean you're in the clear. Restaurant salads can be higher in calories than a cheeseburger and fries, topping out at 1,000 calories and a day's worth of sodium. Don't bother with light salad dressings. They often make up for the lower calories by overloading the sugar, salt, artificial sweeteners, and preservatives. Ask for regular dressing and cheese on the side so you can control calories and prevent a good idea from turning into a fat one.

Make the right swaps. It's not enough to know to avoid added sugars and highly-processed foods. You still have to eat! Knowing the right swaps to make can help you enjoy similar flavors without the negative impact on your body. For example, have a homemade sparkling pomegranate tea over ice (pomegranate tea brewed in 1 cup sparkling water) instead of a Mountain Dew Code Red and you'll save 37 and 38 grams of carbs and sugar, respectively, and 133 calories. For more healthier swaps, see the Appendix and visit EatThis.com.

BEST CARBS
FOR WEIGHT LOSS

Acorn Squash

Besides serving up a third of the day's fiber, a 1-cup serving of this highly nutritious, naturally sweet veggie contains 30 percent of your daily vitamin C needs.

Apples

This fruit provides one of the best and easiest-to-get sources of fiber. A recent study at Wake Forest Baptist Medical Center found that for every 10-gram increase in soluble fiber eaten per day, belly fat was reduced by 3.7 percent over 5 years. And a study at the University of Western Australia found that the Pink Lady variety had the highest level of antioxidant flavonoids—a fat-burning compound—of any apple.

Bananas

This fruit that comes in its own wrapper boosts bloat-fighting bacteria in your stomach and is a prime source of potassium, which can help diminish water retention. Each medium banana contains about 36 grams of good carbs: Their low glycemic index means carbs are slowly released into your body, preventing sugar crashes and spurring muscle recovery.

Barley

Barley is a terrific appetite suppressant because it contains 6 grams of belly-filling, mostly soluble fiber that has been linked to lowered cholesterol, decreased blood sugars and increased satiety. It also has tons of health benefits like decreased inflammation and stabilized blood sugar levels.

Black Beans

Beans are a great source of protein that includes fiber, which means they keep your blood sugar from spiking and provide the building blocks of muscle growth. One cup of black beans has 12 grams of protein and 9 grams of fiber; they're also rich in folate, a B vitamin that stokes muscle growth, and copper, which strengthens tendons. On top of that, a Spanish study showed that consuming four weekly servings of beans or legumes accelerates weight loss.

Legumes

Lentils, chickpeas, peas, and beans—they're all magic bullets for belly-fat loss. In one 4-week Spanish study, researchers found that eating a calorie-restricted diet that includes four weekly servings of legumes aids weight loss more effectively than an equivalent diet that doesn't include them. Those who consumed the legume-rich diet also saw improvements in their "bad" LDL cholesterol levels and systolic blood pressure.

Quinoa

Quinoa is higher in protein than any other grain, and it packs a hefty dose of heart-healthy, unsaturated fats and B vitamins. Try quinoa in the morning. It has twice the protein of most cereals, and fewer carbs.

Sweet Potatoes

Sweet potatoes can be called the king of slow carbs because they're digested slowly and keep you feeling fuller and energized longer, plus they are loaded with fiber, nutrients and can help you burn fat. The magic ingredients here are carotenoids, antioxidants that stabilize blood sugar levels and lower insulin resistance, which prevents calories from being converted into fat. And their high vitamin profile (including A, C and B_6) gives you more energy to burn at the gym.

Tart Cherries

In most of the country you'll find them dried, frozen or canned. But they're worth seeking out because they are a true superpower fruit. Animal studies at the University of Michigan have found that tart cherries have the power to reduce belly fat and alter the expression of fat genes.

Whole-Wheat Bread

You know brown is better, but do you know why? It's because whole wheat contains three parts of the grain, all nutrient rich and full of fiber. Just be careful—most breads in the bread aisle are filled with high-fructose corn syrup or a blend of whole and enriched wheats. It's worth splurging on the pricier stuff, often found in the freezer section.

Whole-Wheat Pasta

As with whole-wheat bread, you're getting all three parts of the grain, with fiber to increase satiety and prevent overeating. For variety, try pastas made from lentils, chickpeas, black beans or quinoa; all are full of fiber.

Yogurt

Packed with protein and probiotics, a cup of yogurt will satisfy hunger and improve your gut health, a key factor in weight loss. It is also rich in vitamin D and calcium, and it's one of the few foods containing conjugated linoleic acid, a special fat that studies show may reduce body fat. But you need to get the right kind to take advantage of these benefits. Most yogurts are full of sugar and fruity sweeteners. Shop for plain Greek yogurt.

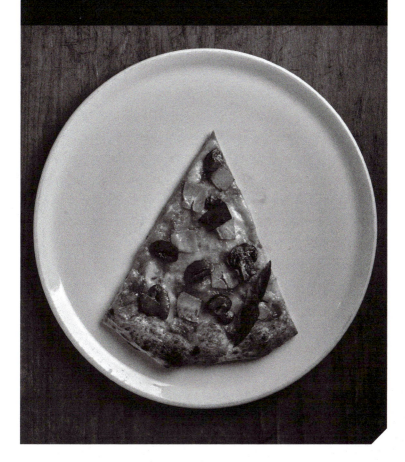

Chapter 3

A Thinner Crust

Made right, pizza dough can be part of a well-rounded diet

Gluten gets a bad rap. In recent years, it's become the most vilified component of our food this side of high-fructose corn syrup.

And while it may be trendy to say you're going gluten-free, the truth of the matter is, unless you're among the 1 percent of the population with celiac disease, gluten may not be your enemy.

Humans have been eating flour for thousands of years, and it's no exaggeration to say that the discovery of the milling process is probably one of the most important innovations in history. It helped build civilization and led to an increased life span for our ancient ancestors.

Flour is not necessarily the problem, but the way we prepare it may be. Like so much in our modern world, industrialization may have stolen what was originally good about our food.

Bread has a pretty simple ingredient list: flour, water, salt, and beginning more than 5,000 years ago, a leavening agent, such as yeast. It's not clear how yeast came to be introduced into bread, but it most likely occurred by accident, and what those long-ago bakers noticed was that its addition caused the bread to rise, making it lighter and fluffier.

What they didn't know back then is what we know now—that the introduction of yeast to the dough not only changes its texture, it changes its chemical makeup.

When we add yeast to dough, the yeast begins eating the sugar in the flour, releasing carbon dioxide as a by-product (which makes your dough puff up). The fermentation process also breaks down the gluten protein into smaller pieces, making it easier for our bodies to digest and increasing its nutritional value. Think of it this way: Fermentation does part of the job of your digestive system: the gluten is being broken down before it even enters your stomach, so all you have to do is take its nutrition once it arrives. Fermentation also lowers bread's glycemic index number, meaning it will be less likely to raise your blood sugar. This is critical because frequent blood sugar spikes can trigger insulin resistance, a precursor to type 2 diabetes and more immediately, cause cravings and extreme hunger when it dips.

Long ago, bread was different. Simpler. It wasn't made from highly processed flour, and it didn't roll out of giant factories, presliced. It was made more carefully, often with a sourdough starter, and allowed to rise for many hours, if not days. Only in the 20th century have new industrial baking techniques made it possible to churn out a loaf ready to eat in about 3 hours.

Bread—and pizza crust—wasn't meant to be produced this way. We've sacrificed speed for nutrition, and we're doing our bodies harm in the process of making baking more profitable. Celiac disease—intolerance of gluten—is now about four times more prevalent than it was 50 years ago, and doctors aren't quite sure why. One theory suggests it may have to do with the quickie, industrialized bread-making techniques and the way that gluten is not sufficiently broken down before it's eaten.

Celiac disease is caused by an abnormal immune-system response to gluten that can damage the lining of the small intestine. The damage can often hinder absorption of nutrients. Sometimes the symptoms are obvious—diarrhea, anemia, bone pain, and a severe skin rash with the scary name of *dermatitis herpetiformis*. Often, however, celiac disease presents no symptoms at all. As a result, only about 5 to 10 percent of cases are diagnosed correctly in the United States. In some cases, those who think they're gluten intolerant might just be intolerant to the overly refined wheat that's so prevalent in America. And many times, those who can't tolerate wheat gluten are able to tolerate other grains that contain gluten, such as kamut, for example.

Demand for wheat has exploded over the years, forcing industrial farming companies to create new strains of the plant and new ways to increase the yield. Monsanto operates a so-called Wheat Technology Center. Personally, I'd prefer my wheat to have as little to do with technology as possible. And what are these new types of wheat, and the pesticides that go with them, doing to our bodies? We don't yet know for sure, but it could be that they're responsible for this seeming rise in celiac disease.

Stress, believe it or not, can also cause gluten intolerance. So how do you know if you actually suffer from celiac disease or if your issue is due to work stress? The only way to know for sure is to undergo a battery of tests. Those who have celiac disease should probably steer clear of gluten, but what about those who don't?

Gluten-free has become a trendy diet fad, and these days, the supermarket shelves are stocked with all sorts of products piously proclaiming their lack of gluten. Sales of these products grew 34 percent annually from 2009 to 2014, and total sales are predicted to reach a massive $2.34 billion in 2019, according to *Packaged Facts*. And the reason for the booming sales is that consumers believe these products are more healthful.

But are they? Not exactly. They're often loaded with starch, which acts very similarly to sugar in the digestive system. A gluten-free diet can also lead to nutritional deficiencies, such as a lack of B vitamins, calcium, iron, zinc, magnesium, and fiber.

Following diets that shun gluten, such as paleo, may not be a healthy alternative. A 2014 study published in the journal *Cell Metabolism* found that people in middle age who ate a diet high in animal protein were four times more likely to die of cancer than those who ate a low-protein diet. Deciding to arbitrarily go gluten-free might not just hit you in the gut; it could hit you in the wallet. A 2007 survey found that the gluten-free products cost twice as much as conventional ones.

> # HOW I LOST 100 POUNDS
>
> Getting the cookies and cakes out of my sight helped me control overeating. I would eat 10 Oreos, sometimes a whole box. It was like a drug for me. But if it wasn't right in front of me, I didn't crave it.

In short, it's time to embrace pizza—even if you're someone who is sensitive to gluten. I've had numerous customers who claim to be gluten intolerant come to my restaurant, eat my pizza and have no ill effects. They claim it's the only pizza they can eat. They might be on to something.

In 2011, the medical journal *Clinical Gastroenterology and Hepatology* published a study involving a group of people who suffered from celiac disease. The subjects were split into three groups and fed bread that had been fermented for different amounts of time. And guess what happened? The people who ate the regular or only mildly fermented bread got sick—some so much that they had to drop out of the study. The patients who ate the highly fermented bread reported "no clinical complaints." In other words, gluten-free people were able to eat gluten if it was prepared in the right way.

This is what I believe. This is what I've discovered in my own life. You do not need to cut pizza out of your life. When the dough is prepared the right way, it can be good for you and part of a well-rounded diet. You'll learn how to do just that in chapter 5.

Chapter 4

Setting the Table

How to prepare for success on the Pizza Diet

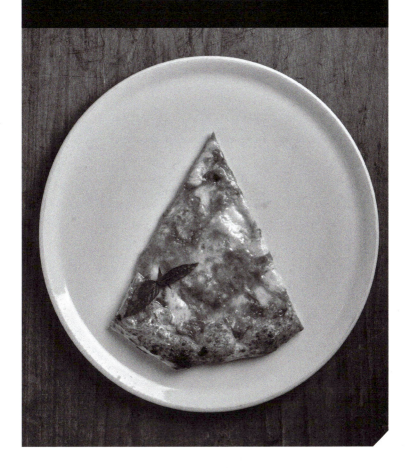

So you're ready to do this? Ready to dive in, start eating pizza every day and still shed pounds? It's possible, and you can do it. But you're going to need to do a few things first.

STEP 1: Set a Goal

There's no point in embarking on this (or any) journey if you don't have a destination in mind. Ask yourself, what are you hoping to accomplish? Do you want to lose 5 pounds or 55? Trim down so you put less pressure on your joints and have less knee pain, for example? Just trying to eat healthier? Decide exactly what it is you want before you get started. And write it down so you can refer to it often.

STEP 2: Pay Your Doctor a Visit

It's not a bad idea to get a checkup to see exactly how healthy you are. A doctor's appointment was a wake-up call for me, and it provided the motivation for me to find a way to lose weight. It was my first step toward eventually developing the Pizza Diet and turning my health around. I highly recommend seeing your doctor.

In addition to your weight and cholesterol levels, determine your body mass index and your basal metabolic rate (BMR), which is basically the amount of energy your body requires to keep running its vital systems while you're at rest. Everyone is different and will require a different number of calories throughout the day. Knowing your BMR and other health information is going to help you better tailor this diet to your specific needs. You might also ask your doctor about a blood sugar test to make sure you aren't prediabetic.

STEP 3: Visualize Positive Changes

How is your life going to be different after you lose weight and accomplish your goals? Think about anyone who might have made fun of you when you were fat, how hard it was sometimes to buy clothes in your size. Think about how guilty you felt when you ate junk food you knew was terrible for you.

There are better things ahead.

Once you get your old body back, you're going to have more energy and feel better. You may be able to play sports and take part in other activities that you now find challenging. For me, I visualized that moment when I'd be able to fit into my old clothes again. Before I started the Pizza Diet, I went to the store and picked out a pair of jeans that were intentionally much smaller than I could fit into. They were size 42—the size I wore as a young man before I packed on all those pounds. At the time, though, I was wearing size 60. I didn't hide those size-42 pants away in the closet in a drawer. I kept them out in plain view to remind myself what I was working toward and to assure myself that one day I would fit into them. Nine months later, I did.

STEP 4: Clean Out Your Kitchen

It's going to be painful, but grab a trash bag or two and start cleaning out all the unhealthy food and ingredients from your home. You probably already know what they are. Is it processed packaged food? Get rid of it. Is it nothing but a vehicle for empty calories? Gone. Does it have the words "double stuff"in the title? Toss it.

Get rid of all the junk food, all those bags of chips and cookies. Toss out that jar of mayonnaise and those bags of worthless white flour. Go through your fridge and cabinets and remove it all. You can't be tempted to eat it if it's not there. Plus, you need to make room for all the healthy items you'll be bringing in. A couple months into this diet, and you won't even crave that junk food anymore. You won't want it, even if it's offered to you or in reach. But for now, get cleaning.

STEP 5: Buy The Good Stuff

It's time to fill that space in your kitchen that you created by throwing away all those bags of Doritos with something else. There are two parts to your resupply plan. First, stock up on the foundation foods of the Mediterranean style of eating: fresh produce, fish, whole grains, and healthy fats. Make a habit of shopping the perimeter of your grocery store where the healthiest foods are found, and shop seasonally at farm stands for fresh, locally grown vegetables, fruits, cheeses and meats. Use the grocery shopping list that starts on 55 as a guide.

Secondly, include on your shopping list the key ingredients for making your pizzas, including the toppings for your pies. Make sure you stock up on plenty of the staples: sea salt, canned San Marzano tomatoes, yeast and the Italian-style flour you'll be using to make the pizza dough. (More on that in chapter 5.) It's difficult to find at the corner grocery, so you may want to buy it online well in advance. You'll also need high-quality extra-virgin olive oil (EVOO). The olive oil world can be confusing, and trying to pick one out can seem as daunting as trying to select a suitable Pinot Noir at the wine store. The store shelves are often packed with literally dozens of varieties, and unfortunately, the olive oil industry is rife with fraud. Some bottles labeled EVOO are really just cheaper oils, such as sunflower, that have been adulterated to look and smell like olive oil.

The most important safeguard is to read the label and see where the oil was produced. Make sure it says it's made in Italy from Italian olives. Some oils are just packed in Italy, meaning they're bottled there using fruit from other places, such as Spain. Also look for a "sell-by" date. Olive oil is basically the juice of the olive, and like real fruit juice, it's perishable. If it doesn't have a date on the label, don't buy it.

Now, depending on how you plan to cook the pizza, you may require a few new kitchen gadgets. For conventional oven baking, get a pizza stone. The name says it all—it's a circular cooking aid made of stone (or sometimes ceramic) that's placed inside your oven, and your pizza is cooked atop it in lieu of a baking sheet. The porous nature of the stone retains heat, allowing the pizza to cook more evenly, and it absorbs moisture in the pizza dough, resulting in a crispier crust. Pizza stones are available on Amazon, and at specialty kitchen supply stores such as Williams-Sonoma or Bed Bath & Beyond, for between $15 and $50.

Caring for Your Pizza Stone

Never wash your stone with soap because the pores will absorb the soap and make your next pizza taste like Palmolive.

You don't even need water to clean your stone. Simply scrape off the baked-on cheese with a pizza stone scrubber, a stiff, non-metal brush or a plastic scraper. Tomato sauce stains add character (and flavor), so don't worry about making it look like new.

You can also bypass your oven altogether and instead buy a countertop electric pizza oven. They're available, often for under $100, on Amazon and other online stores, and they really do work.

If you plan to cook your pizza in advance and heat it up at the office for lunch, consider buying a toaster oven. Your office kitchen probably has a microwave, but a toaster oven will give you much better results when it comes to reheating. (Make sure to ban your coworker from using it to cook her stinky fish.) Inexpensive models are available for under $25.

For many of my dinner recipes, you're going to need a stove-top grill pan. They're great for cooking protein simply without any added oil. Ikea offers one (creatively called the Grilla) for around $25. And one last thing you're going to need: A scale to weigh yourself.

STEP 6: Plan Your Meals

I like to draw up my meals for the next 15 days, but a week is fine, as well. What's important is that you know what you need to have on hand, and there will be no doubts about what you're eating each day. The tighter the plan, the less likely you are to stray from it, say, by popping into Taco Bell because you realized you didn't have anything in the house for dinner.

Write down every breakfast, lunch and dinner, plus snacks, for the upcoming week and shop for it at once. You will also want to figure out exactly when and how you're going to eat your pizza. I have mine every day for lunch, but I realize it's unrealistic for those with certain kinds of jobs (construction worker, taxi driver) to whip up a fresh pie in the middle of the day. You're welcome to have the pizza for dinner instead. For lunch, just eat something that falls within the parameters of this plan.

THE PIZZA DIET

You can also bake a few completely assembled pies according to my recipes, let them cool, then seal them in a plastic bag and freeze. In the morning before you head out to work, school or wherever you're going, grab the pizza out of the freezer and come lunchtime, reheat it.

Pizza dough freezes well, so you have the option of making a week's worth on a Sunday and just pulling the dough balls out of the freezer as you need them. The other option is to make it fresh every 3 days. Just remember, because of the long fermentation time, you're going to have to prepare it at least a day and a half before you plan to bake it. It can sit in the refrigerator for up to 3 days after it's first made, but no longer.

And lastly, try and make time for family dinners. Eat with others around the same table, the way Italian families do. It's a way to talk about your day, and it creates a sense that food is life. It's also a good way to share your weight-loss progress with your loved ones and to keep you motivated.

STEP 7: Start Drinking More Water

It's always a good idea to stay hydrated, no matter what you're doing. But when you're dieting, it's even better. Drinking the proper amount of water could keep you feeling full and help you avoid overeating. Many confuse thirst with hunger and reach for a snack instead of a glass of H_2O. I try to drink at least a half gallon of water each day.

STEP 8: Stop Sitting Around

This diet is already magical enough in that it allows you to eat pizza every day, but it's not so magical that it doesn't require some sort of exercise to see better results. Join a gym, if you can. Start exercising regularly. If nothing else, try and work out for 10 to 15 minutes each morning, doing sit-ups, push-ups and pull-ups. Or walk briskly for 25 minutes during the day. It's time to get up and get moving.

Save 50 Calories!

When you see a pool of oil floating on top of your cheese, take a napkin and mop up the excess. You'll save about 50 calories ... and maybe keep the grease off your shirt!

Once you've completed these steps, you'll be on your way. Don't be afraid to start changing your life. Remember, you'll be following a meal plan that allows you eat some of your favorite foods, including pizza. This is not only doable, you should wake up each day, as I do, knowing there's a delicious pizza waiting for you. This might not even feel like a diet. But if you really start craving something that's not on the plan—that's what the cheat day is for.

SIX EASY SLICES
Smart Ways to Cut Calories from Takeout Pizza

Yes, you can eat pizzeria pizza on occasion and still follow the Pizza Diet. Just follow these simple tricks for keeping calories from getting out of hand when you do.

Don't Be Plain: You can lower any pizzeria pizza's Glycemic Index (GI)—a measure of how quickly blood glucose levels rise in response to a certain food—by adding fiber- and protein-rich toppings. For example, while a simple cheese pizza scores an 80 out of 100 on the GI scale, a veggie supreme pie clocks in at 49. Raw veggies and lean meats (chicken breast, ham) make for the best toppers for lowering GI. You can further escape sodium and fat overload by keeping processed meats like bacon and sausage off your pie. Watch out for veggies, too, which are often cooked in a bath of oil!

See Red: The biggest health benefits from pizza come from lycopene-rich tomato sauce, which recent studies have found may help protect against the development of prostate cancer. White pizzas sacrifice the biggest health benefit of a traditional pie, so think like Quentin Tarantino: the more red the better.

Think Thin: Most of the evils of pizza lay in the empty-calorie, yet highly caloric crust, typically made from refined white flour. Pizza dough offers little nutrition to your body and will spike your insulin levels, causing you to crave more. That's the difference between my pizzas and other pizzas. As

I mentioned earlier, I use specially made dough that limits the impact on your blood sugar. But you can't always find that dough at pizzerias. So, at restaurants, try to keep the dough to a minimum. The less crust you indulge in, the better. That means thin-crust pizzas are almost always the better option.

Cut the Cheese: Ordering your pizza with "half cheese" is an easy way to cut the saturated fat on a plain- or vegetable-topped pie by 50 percent! Even if you decide to boost the cheese factor on your slimmed-down pie with an additional tablespoon of pungent Parmesan (only 22 calories), you'll still save a lot of calories.

Turn up the Heat: You can trick yourself into eating less and boost your metabolism by adding a little spice to your pie. In fact, a study by Canadian researchers found that men who ate spicy appetizers consumed 200 fewer calories than those that skipped the hot sauce. Top your pie with a few grinds of fresh black pepper, red chile flakes, or if you're really brave—stingers.

Go Green: A series of well-cited Yale University studies suggest eating a salad appetizer can reduce total calorie intake over the course of the meal by up to 20 percent. So when ordering at a restaurant, start the meal with a big garden salad. Top your greens with a scant tablespoon of vinaigrette. Developing research suggests vinegar can aid weight loss by keeping our blood sugar steady. One study among pre-diabetics found the addition of vinegar to a high-carb meal (like pizza!) reduced the subsequent rise in blood sugar by 34 percent.

YOUR PIZZA DIET GROCERY LIST
KEEP HEALTHY FOODS HANDY BY SHOPPING RIGHT

EVERYDAY FOODS

FRUITS:

apples	oranges
apricots	peaches
bananas	pears
blueberries	plums
cherries	pomegranates
figs	raspberries
lemons	strawberries
mangoes	dried fruits

VEGETABLES:

acorn squash	green onions
artichokes	kale
arugula	leeks
asparagus	lettuce
avocado	mushrooms
beets	mustard greens
bell peppers	olives
broccoli	onions
broccoli rabe	peas
Brussels sprouts	potatoes

carrots

celery

celery root

cucumber

eggplant

endive

fennel

garlic

green beans

pumpkin

shallots

spinach

sugar snap peas

Swiss chard

tomatoes

turnips

zucchini

GRAINS:

mostly whole and cracked

barley

bulgur wheat

farro

oats

polenta

quinoa

rice

whole-grain breads

whole-grain tortillas

whole-wheat couscous

whole-wheat flour

whole-wheat pasta

BEANS AND LEGUMES:

black beans

black-eyed peas

cannellini beans

chickpeas

fava beans

lentils

lima beans

white beans

NUTS, SEEDS, AND NUT BUTTERS:

almonds	pine nuts
coconut	sesame seeds
flaxseeds	sunflower seeds
hazelnuts	tahini
pecans	walnuts

OILS:

olive oil	peanut oil

HERBS:

basil	mint
bay leaves	oregano
chives	parsley
cilantro	rosemary
dill	tarragon
herbes de Provence	thyme
marjoram	

SPICES:

allspice	cumin
baharat	fennel seeds
cardamom	garlic powder
cayenne	ginger
chile flakes	Italian seasoning
chipotle chile	nutmeg
cinnamon	paprika

cloves

coriander

saffron

turmeric

TWICE-A-WEEK FOODS

SEAFOOD:

anchovies

bluefish

cod

flounder

halibut

monkfish

salmon

sardines

sea bass

tuna

SHELLFISH:

clams

mussels

shrimp

lobster

CONDIMENTS AND PANTRY

almond milk

baking powder

baking soda

unsweetened cocoa powder

vanilla extract

arrowroot

broth

capers

hummus

mustard

tomato paste

vinegar (e.g., apple cider vinegar, balsamic vinegar, red wine vinegar)

OCCASIONAL FOODS

chicken thighs

lean ground beef

pork

flank steak

turkey breast

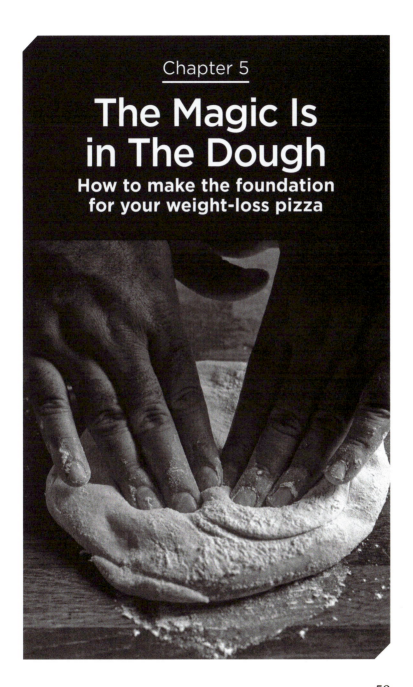

Chapter 5

The Magic Is in The Dough

How to make the foundation for your weight-loss pizza

When I tell other chefs how I make my pizza, the reaction I usually get is, "You're crazy!" And this in New York City, a town where chorizo ice cream is on the menu.

It's true, my method takes a lot more time and costs a bit more, but I think it's worth it.

The secret is the dough. I make it the way it was made many years ago in Italy before the technique was abandoned in favor of cheaper, less labor-intensive ways. These days, people roll out of bed, go to 3 weeks of pizza training and think they're a pizza baker. But it's not just the recipe. You have to understand the chemistry of baking.

I have a lot of passion for my job, and because I'm curious, I like to discover new techniques. It took me nearly 3 years to come up with my recipe for healthier pizza dough. It started when I met a man who worked at a famous Italian flour company in Italy. He was an old guy, very knowledgeable, and he opened my mind. He told me there's another way to make pizza.

In short, use a better quality of flour, and you'll get a better result. So I started experimenting. It was 2013.

In Italy, flour is classified into four main types—2, 1, 0 and 00—according to the way it's produced and how finely it's milled. Type 2 is the coarsest, and type 00 the finest.

You may have heard of type 00 flour. It's the Italian type commonly used for fresh pasta and pizza dough, and chances are, you will find a bag in every corner grocery store and pizzeria. It's as common as red-checked tablecloths.

But it's also the most highly refined variety of flour and not necessarily the most nutritious. The milling process strips it of nearly all of its bran, as well as its vitamins and minerals. It's very similar to American white flour, which is so nutritionally deficient, the government requires it to be enriched with iron, vitamin B and other things that were lost during the harsh refining process.

For many years, I used 00 flour because everyone else did. But then I started to learn more about nutrition, and I made a change that makes my pizza far more nourishing and something you can build a healthy diet around.

For the pizza at my restaurant Ribalta in New York City, I use type 1 stone-milled flour from an Italian maker called Le 5 Stagioni. It's a beautiful product, but unfortunately is not widely available at the retail level in the U.S.; however, you can find it on Amazon. (Look for the bag labeled "Tipo 1.") A good alternative, also available online, is Molino Rossetto's "Grano Duro Cappelli—Farina Macinata a Pietra."

Stone-ground flour, which is literally made by pulverizing the grain between two heavy stones, is more expensive to produce, and that's one reason why many restaurants don't use it. One 50-pound bag of 00 flour imported from Italy will run $27. A bag of the stone-ground will cost me $37.

The flour you'll be using is better for your body, but the biggest difference between my pizza—the pizza you will be eating on this diet—and regular pizza is the raising time. As I wrote in chapter 3, dough needs to be fermented for a long time in order for the yeast to go to work and the gluten to be adequately broken down.

I allow my dough to rise for at least 36 hours. That's a full day and a half. Generally, other pizzerias might let their dough rise for no more than 5 hours. It ends up heavy, like a rock in your stomach. No wonder you fall into a food coma after you eat a slice.

My process costs a bit more. From a business perspective, it doesn't make the most sense, but my customers tell me over and over again that they can taste the difference. My pizza is lighter; it melts in your mouth. Customers claim that they could eat two of them at one sitting.

Your average corner pizza place doesn't do it my way because it takes training to learn to make pizza this special way, and getting your staff up to speed is expensive.

Fermenting your dough also requires space—lots of it. At Ribalta, I make dough three times a day and store up to 600 balls in a large walk-in refrigerator, where they can slowly ferment at 42°F.

Regular pizzerias are about volume and turnover. They're looking to sell a slice quickly and cheaply, sometimes for as low as 99 cents. They often don't have the time or the space to store large amounts of dough and let it rise. They frequently don't have the knowledge either, having been taught the quick and dirty way to make their product.

When you make the dough according to my recipe, here are some of the advantages.

MORE VITAMINS AND MINERALS

Despite its wholesome reputation, white flour is one of the most nutritionally deficient substances you can put into your body. Everything that was once healthy in the wheat kernel gets stripped away in the lengthy refining and bleaching process. It has virtually no fiber, and more than 100 vitamins are also removed. By using a better type of flour, you give your body more of the fiber and vitamins that are lost with white or 00 flour. Studies have shown that we absorb vitamins and minerals better from fermented bread than nonfermented.

EASIER TO DIGEST

The long fermentation process breaks down the bread's gluten, allowing our bodies to properly digest it. It might even be possible for those who are gluten intolerant to follow this diet.

LESS BLOATING

That distended belly and uncomfortable feeling you get after eating some pizza may not be all in your head. Research suggests that when bread doesn't get fermented before you eat it, your body is forced to break it down in your belly, producing gas and bloating.

LOWER GLYCEMIC INDEX

The particles in stone-ground flour are larger than those in flour made by the traditional industrial method. It's harder to digest, which is actually a good thing, as it's slower to absorb into our bloodstream and leads to a smaller spike in blood sugar.

RECIPES FOR
PIZZA DIET DOUGH VARIETIES

Making dough right takes time. You don't want to have to do it daily. So the following recipes are designed to make enough for at least a week's worth. Keep the dough refrigerated until ready to use. Or double the recipes and freeze half for another week.

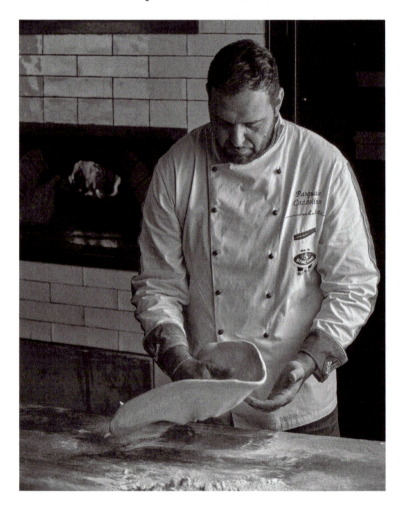

PIZZA DIET TRADITIONAL DOUGH

(makes eleven 12-inch pizzas)

35 oz cold water

1 tsp dry yeast

3.65 lb Italian stone-ground flour

3 Tbsp sea salt

Pour the water into a large mixing bowl and add the yeast. Mix with your hands, breaking up the clumps of yeast. Let stand for 5 minutes until all the yeast has dissolved.

Add 20 percent of the flour (about ½ cup) and mix with your hands until a creamy slurry forms.

Add the salt and the remaining flour and mix by hand (or use a stand mixer) until a soft, elastic dough has formed.

Transfer to a floured work surface and knead and fold with your hands for 5 minutes. If the dough is too wet, add a bit more flour.

Cover with plastic wrap and allow the dough to rest at room temperature for 20 minutes.

Cut the dough into balls of about 8 ounces each. Seal in an airtight container and let rest for 4 or 5 hours at room temperature. Move into the refrigerator and let rise for another 20 hours. You can let it rise for longer, but no more than 48 hours, as it will begin to sour. Dough can be frozen for up to 6 months.

PIZZA DIET GLUTEN-FREE DOUGH

(makes 5 to 6 pizzas)

3½ cups gluten-free flour (could be an equal mix of potato, corn and rice flours)

2 Tbsp extra-virgin olive oil

2 Tbsp + 1 tsp brewer's yeast

1 Tbsp sea salt (if there's no added salt in the flour)

2 cups water

In a large bowl, mix all the ingredients together.

Let rise for 2 hours at room temperature.

When shaping the dough to make pizzas, use caution, as it's more delicate and prone to breaking.

PIZZA DIET WHOLE-WHEAT DOUGH

(makes eleven 12-inch pizzas)

37 oz cold water

1 tsp dry yeast

3.65 lb stone-ground, whole-wheat flour

3 Tbsp sea salt

Pour the water into a large mixing bowl and add the yeast.

Mix with your hands, breaking up the clumps of yeast.

Let stand for 5 minutes until all the yeast has dissolved.

Add 20 percent of the flour and mix with your hands until a creamy slurry forms.

Add the salt and the remaining flour and mix by hand (or use a stand mixer) until a soft, elastic dough has formed.

Transfer to a floured work surface and knead and fold with your hands for 5 minutes. If the dough is too wet, add a bit more flour.

Cover with plastic wrap and allow the dough to rest at room temperature for 20 minutes.

Cut the dough into balls of about 8 ounces each. Seal in an airtight container and let rest for 4 or 5 hours at room temperature. Move into the refrigerator and let rise for another 20 hours. You can let it rise for longer, but no more than 48 hours, as it will begin to sour. Dough can be frozen for up to 6 months.

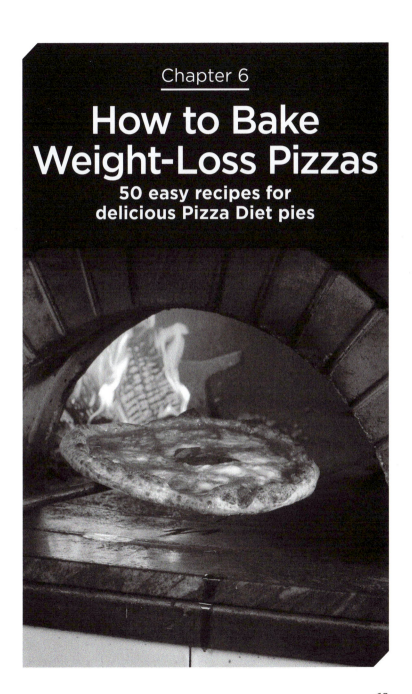

Chapter 6

How to Bake Weight-Loss Pizzas

50 easy recipes for delicious Pizza Diet pies

This is it—the main event. It's time to make the pizza. The dough, which we discussed in the last chapter, is a critical component, but so are the toppings. Aim to use the highest-quality, most natural ingredients you can find.

And no matter how much you love pizza, no one wants to eat the same kind every day. What follows are recipes for 50 different varieties that should keep you from getting bored for months or even years. Or feel free to invent your own.

The red sauce for these recipes is simple to make. Empty one 14-ounce can of whole, peeled San Marzano tomatoes into a bowl, add two generous pinches of sea salt, then crush by hand into a chunky pulp. Keep a stock in your refrigerator for the week.

I always use fresh mozzarella cheese, preferably from a local maker. Don't even think about buying that bagged, shredded stuff. It's often loaded with preservatives and other unappetizing additives, including wood pulp. Three 8-ounce balls of cheese should be enough for the 11 pizzas that the dough recipe makes. Simply take the ball of cheese and pull off 1-inch chunks when you're ready to make your pizza.

Three quick notes:

If you're planning to freeze whole pies to reheat later, follow the recipes to the end, then allow the pizza to completely cool before sealing it in a Ziploc bag. To reheat, remove from the freezer and the bag. Bake at 500°F for 6 to 7 minutes. It can be reheated after it's been thawed, as well. It makes no difference in taste or texture.

Also, each single-serve recipe uses an 8-ounce ball of dough, and it should be prepped the same way, unless specifically instructed in the recipe. Remove the dough ball from the refrigerator and allow to rest at room temperature for 1 hour. On a floured surface, flatten the dough with your fingertips and palm, starting at the center and working outward until you have a 12-inch disc. Leave ½ inch around the edge unflattened for the crust.

Finally, never top the raw dough with hot ingredients. Some of these recipes require you to cook meat and other toppings before you place them atop your pie. Always allow your precooked toppings to cool to room temperature before adding. They'll melt the dough and ruin your pizza.

HOW I LOST 100 POUNDS

Start a meal with a glass of water, a soup or salad, even a piece of fruit, anything with high water content or fiber to fill you up. Sometimes I didn't have to finish the pizza. I was satisfied.

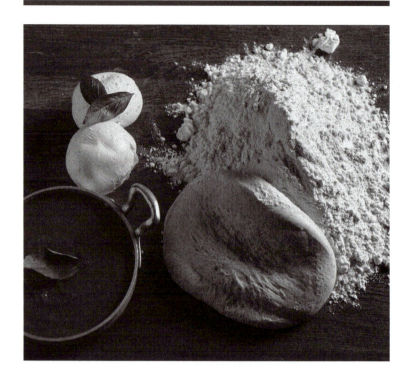

THE PIZZA PROCESS
Step-by-Step Instructions
for Making a Leaner, Healthy,
Home-Baked Pizza

Start by gathering your supplies: the dough made with Italian-style Type 1 flour, which has been allowed to rise, canned San Marzano tomatoes, sea salt, mozzarella cheese, high-quality extra-virgin olive oil, and the toppings. Optional but highly recommended: A pizza baking stone.

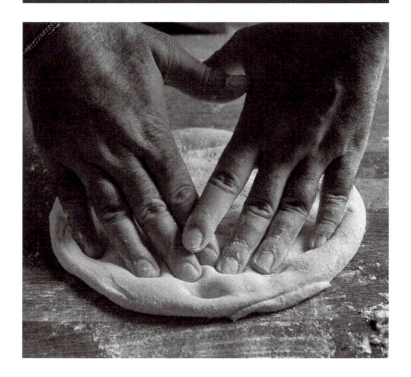

Prepare Your Workspace: Toss some flour on your work surface so the dough won't stick. Your dough has been rising for 24 to 36 hours, right? Great! Now plop the 8-ounce ball of dough down and get to work.

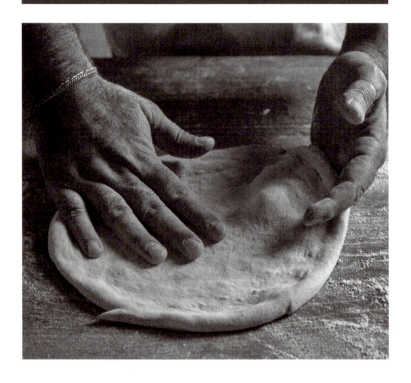

Start Forming Your Base: Press down with your fingertips to flatten it, leaving a thicker rim or cornicione (core-nee-CHO-neh), Italian for "cornice."

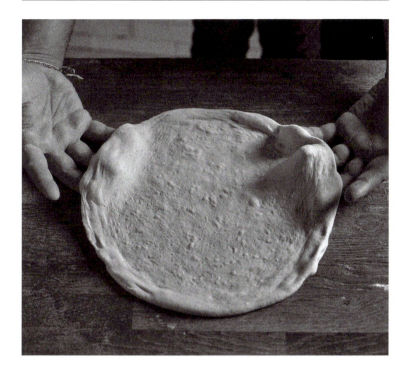

Shoot for Symmetry: Form a circle 12 inches in diameter. Stretch from the rim to avoid making the center too thin and tearing a hole in the dough.

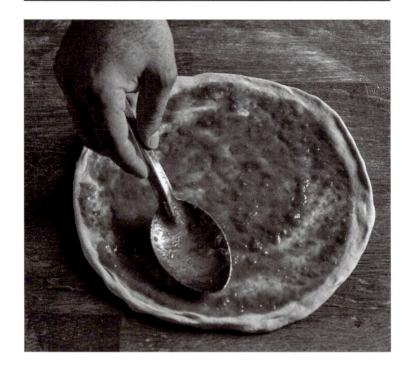

Spread the Sauce: Spoon a ladle of tomato sauce (about 3 table-spoons) into the center of your dough. Using the rounded back of the spoon, carefully circle your pie to spread the sauce evenly out to the cornicione edge.

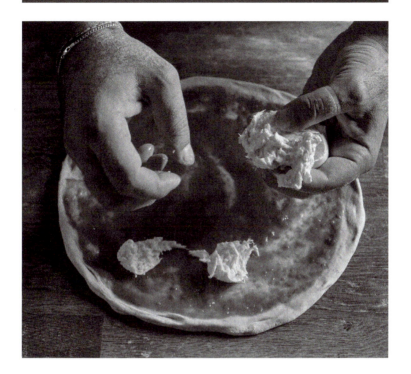

Chunk the Cheese: Don't slice the cheese. Instead, pull one-inch chunks off a fresh roll of local mozzarella cheese and arrange them evenly on top of the tomato sauce.

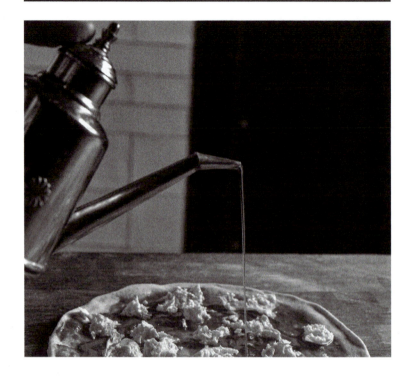

Add a Touch of EVOO: Drizzle a little extra-virgin olive oil over your creation. Not too much, though, or pools of oil will make your pie a bit soggy.

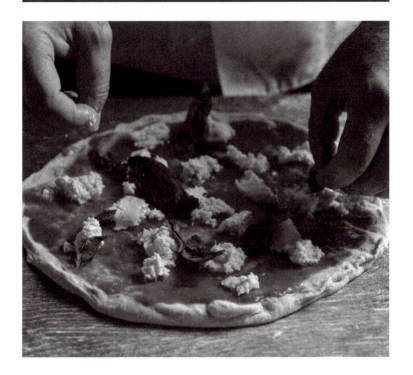

Garnish with Green: Finally, arrange fresh basil leaves over your margherita, which should resemble the colors of the Italian flag. *Fantastico!*

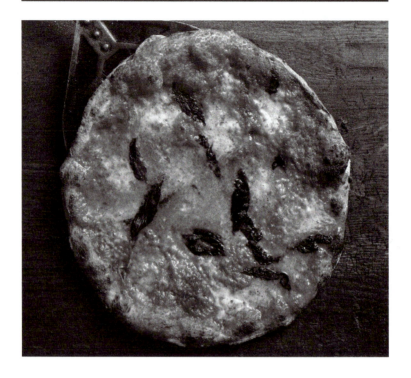

Make it Hot: Preheat an oven to 500°F. Place the pizza on a parchment-lined baking sheet or a pizza stone and bake for 10 to 11 minutes until the crust is golden brown and looks like this. That's your classic Neapolitan margherita.

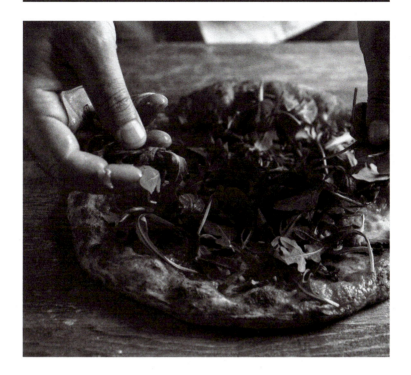

ADD MORE TOPPINGS

Pile On: You can turn your margherita into a more elaborate and nutritious pizza using colorful toppings, starting with a large handful of my favorite, arugula leaves. This tangy green is rich in healthful nutrients like alpha-lipoic acid and sulforaphane, plus calcium and vitamin K.

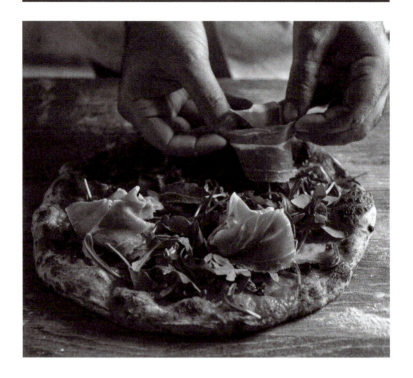

Top with Protein: On top of the greens, arrange thin slices of pro-sciutto di Parma ham, which will add a salty flavor to complement the peppery bite of the arugula.

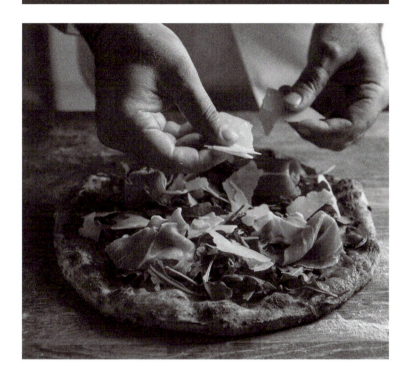

More Cheese, Please: Place large, thinly shaved pieces of Parmiggiano-Reggiano cheese over the toppings.

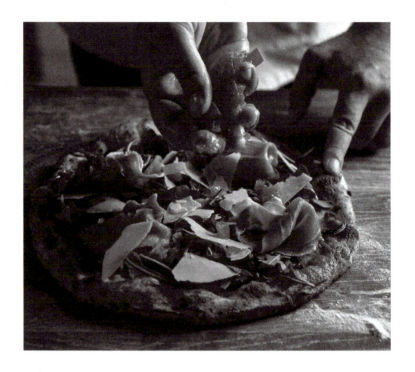

More Color: Finally, add a half-cup or so of diced raw Better Boy tomato on top. *Bellissimo!*

Now, on to more easy Pizza Diet recipes!

ANCHOVY

3 Tbsp tomato sauce

8 oz pizza dough

2 tsp fresh chopped parsley

4–5 anchovy fillets, canned

1 tsp dried oregano

2 oz fresh mozzarella, cubed

4 large basil leaves

1 Tbsp extra-virgin olive oil

Preheat the oven to 500°F.

Place the pizza stone inside, if using.

Spread the tomato sauce on the dough. Top with the parsley, anchovies, oregano, and then the mozzarella and basil leaves. Drizzle with olive oil. Bake on a parchment-lined baking sheet or a pizza stone for 10 to 11 minutes until the crust is golden brown.

Don't forget the humble anchovy

While salmon, tuna, and other big fish get all the kudos for being rich in heart-healthy omega-3 fatty acids, the tiny fish topping this anchovy pizza delivers more than half of the 1,000 milligrams of omega-3s you should get every day.

How to Bake Weight-Loss Pizzas

ARUGULA AND PROSCIUTTO

8 oz pizza dough

3 Tbsp tomato sauce

2 oz fresh mozzarella, cubed

1 Tbsp extra-virgin olive oil

1 generous handful fresh arugula

4 slices proscuitto di Parma

Shaved Parmesan cheese, 4 thin slices broken

½ cup Better Boy tomato, chopped

Preheat the oven to 500°F.

Place the pizza stone inside, if using.

Top the dough with the tomato sauce and mozzarella. Drizzle with olive oil.

Bake on a parchment-lined baking sheet or a pizza stone for 10 to 11 minutes until the crust is golden brown.

Top the pizza with arugula, proscuitto, shaved Parmesan and tomatoes.

ASPARAGUS WITH ARUGULA PESTO

3 stalks fresh asparagus

1 generous handful of fresh arugula

1 tsp extra-virgin olive oil

1.7 oz grated Grana Padano cheese, divided

1 garlic clove, peeled

6–7 pine nuts

8 oz pizza dough

2.5 oz fresh mozzarella, cubed

Preheat the oven to 500°F.

Place the pizza stone inside, if using.

Cook the asparagus over boiling water in a steamer basket for 5 minutes until softened and bright green. (Can also be grilled for 5 minutes.) Slice in half lengthwise.

Rinse the arugula and place in a food processor with 1 teaspoon extra-virgin olive oil, 1 tablespoon Grana Padano, the garlic and the pine nuts. Blend until smooth.

Top the dough with the mozzarella and bake on a parchment-lined baking sheet or a pizza stone for 6 minutes.

Add the asparagus, arranging the spears in a sun-like pattern, and bake for an additional 6 minutes until the crust is golden brown.

Remove from the oven and sprinkle with the remainder of the cheese. Drizzle with the arugula pesto, streaking it across the pizza in lines.

BACCALAU

3.5 oz fresh or frozen Alaskan cod

½ cup water

¼ cup white wine

1 tsp chile flakes

1 onion, thinly sliced

2 tsp fresh chopped parsley

8 oz pizza dough

1 tsp extra-virgin olive oil

Preheat the oven to 500°F.

Place the pizza stone inside, if using.

If the fish is frozen, defrost it first. Bring the water to boil in a pan. Add the cod, white wine, chile flakes, onion and parsley. Cook for 8 minutes, remove from the liquid and break the fish into chunks. Let cool and then place atop the dough. Drizzle the olive oil over the entire pizza.

Bake on a parchment-lined baking sheet or a pizza stone for 10 to 11 minutes until the crust is golden brown.

(Alternatively, this pizza can be made with 3 tablespoons tomato sauce. Simply add it to the crust before the cod, then top with 5 sliced olives and capers.)

BASIL PESTO

1 spoonful of jarred basil pesto

8 oz pizza dough

4 cherry tomatoes, quartered

2 oz fresh mozzarella, cubed

1 tsp extra-virgin olive oil

5 pieces of shaved Pecorino Romano cheese

Preheat the oven to 500°F.

Place the pizza stone inside, if using.

Spread the pesto over the dough. Top with the tomatoes and mozzarella. Drizzle with olive oil.

Bake on a parchment-lined baking sheet or a pizza stone for 14 minutes until golden brown.

Garnish with the Pecorino Romano.

Basil is the Swiss Army knife of herbs

It boasts antioxidant, antiviral, and antibacterial properties and may even inhibit the formation of tumors.

BRESAOLA

8 oz pizza dough

2 oz fresh mozzarella, cubed

1 Tbsp extra-virgin olive oil

2 cups arugula (or as much as you'd like)

6 cherry tomatoes, quartered

4 very thin slices of bresaola

1 Tbsp lemon juice

Preheat the oven to 500°F.

Place the pizza stone inside, if using.

Top the dough with the mozzarella and drizzle with olive oil.

Bake on a parchment-lined baking sheet or a pizza stone for 10 to 11 minutes until the crust is golden brown.

Remove from the oven and top with the arugula, tomatoes and bresaola. Dress with lemon juice and fresh black pepper.

Go ahead, make more dough

To save time, make enough dough for a week's worth of pizzas. You can even make more and freeze some. Before freezing your dough, ball it, wrap it in plastic wrap, and let it sit in the refrigerator for 24 hours.

BROCCOLI

3.5 oz broccoli, cut into florets

2 Tbsp olive oil

1 garlic clove, minced

2 canned anchovy fillets, chopped

8 oz pizza dough

2 oz fresh mozzarella, cubed

Preheat the oven to 500°F.

Place the pizza stone inside, if using.

Wash the broccoli, then boil in salted water until al dente, about 5 minutes.

Drain and sauté in a pan with 1 tablespoon olive oil, the garlic and the anchovies over medium heat, about 5 minutes. Remove from the heat and allow to cool.

Top the dough with the broccoli mixture and mozzarella. Drizzle with olive oil.

Bake on a parchment-lined baking sheet or a pizza stone for 12 minutes until the crust is golden brown.

BROCCOLI RABE

1 bunch broccoli rabe

1 Tbsp extra-virgin olive oil

1 garlic clove, minced

Pinch of chile flakes, to taste

8 oz pizza dough

2 oz fresh mozzarella, cubed

Half of 1 sweet Italian sausage (optional)

Preheat the oven to 500°F.

Place the pizza stone inside, if using.

Boil the broccoli rabe for 5 to 6 minutes. Drain. Sauté with 1 tablespoon olive oil, the garlic, chile flakes and a pinch of sea salt. Remove from the heat and allow to cool.

Top the dough with the broccoli rabe and mozzarella. If this is a cheat day, you may add the sausage. Remove the casing and sprinkle the meat across the pizza.

Bake on a parchment-lined baking sheet or a pizza stone for 14 minutes until golden brown.

BUFFALO MOZZARELLA AND EGGPLANT

1 eggplant, sliced

2 Tbsp tomato sauce

8 oz pizza dough

2 oz fresh buffalo mozzarella

1 Tbsp Parmesan cheese

1 Tbsp extra-virgin olive oil

4 large basil leaves

Preheat the oven to 500°F.

Place the pizza stone inside, if using.

Cook the eggplant on a grill or in a dry grill pan over medium heat for 7 minutes until softened and blackened on the edges. Remove from the heat and allow to cool.

Spread the tomato sauce on the dough. Top with the grilled eggplant, the mozzarella, the Parmesan cheese, extra-virgin olive oil and basil leaves.

Bake on a parchment-lined baking sheet or a pizza stone for 10 to 11 minutes until the crust is golden brown.

BURRATA

3 Tbsp tomato sauce

8 oz pizza dough

2 oz fresh burrata cheese, chopped

4 large basil leaves

1 Tbsp extra-virgin olive oil

4 thin slices of prosciutto di Parma

Preheat the oven to 500°F.

Place the pizza stone inside, if using.

Spread the tomato sauce on the dough. Top with the burrata and basil. Drizzle with olive oil.

Bake on a parchment-lined baking sheet or a pizza stone for 10 to 11 minutes until the crust is golden brown. Remove from the oven and top with prosciutto di Parma.

Drizzle your pizza with healthy fat

Extra-virgin olive oil, a staple of the Mediterranean Diet, is heart healthy not only because monounsaturated fats are better for you than butter and lard, but also because it contains good amounts of powerful antioxidants called polyphenols.

CALZONE ESCAROLE

8 oz pizza dough

1 handful of endive, chopped

1 tsp raisins

4 black olives, sliced

2 canned anchovy fillets, chopped

1 tsp capers

1 tsp extra-virgin olive oil

Preheat the oven to 500°F.

Place the pizza stone inside, if using.

Top one half of the dough with the endive, raisins, olives, anchovies, and capers. Drizzle with olive oil.

Fold the dough over the filling to form a half-moon shape. Seal the edges with your fingers or a fork. Brush the top with a little oil and poke a hole to allow steam to escape.

Bake on a parchment-lined baking sheet or a pizza stone for 14 minutes until golden brown.

CAPRESE

1 Tbsp + 1 tsp extra-virgin olive oil

1 large tomato, sliced

4 large basil leaves, roughly torn

8 oz pizza dough

2 oz fresh mozzarella, cubed

Preheat the oven to 500°F.

Place the pizza stone inside, if using.

Mix 1 teaspoon of the olive oil, the tomato and the basil together. Season with sea salt and pepper.

Drizzle the dough with 1 tablespoon olive oil. Bake on a parchment-lined baking sheet or a pizza stone for 12 minutes until the crust is golden brown.

Remove from the oven and top with the tomato mixture and fresh mozzarella.

How to keep your basil fresh

Don't store basil in the refrigerator; the leaves will discolor. Instead, keep fresh basil ready for your pizzas by placing in a glass of water on the kitchen counter as you would cut flowers.

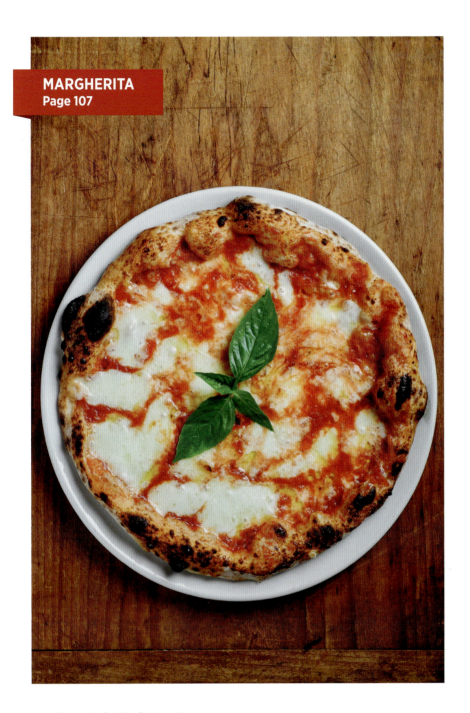

MARGHERITA
Page 107

How to Bake Weight-Loss Pizzas

PERFECT PIZZA STEP-BY-STEP

See detailed instructions on page 72

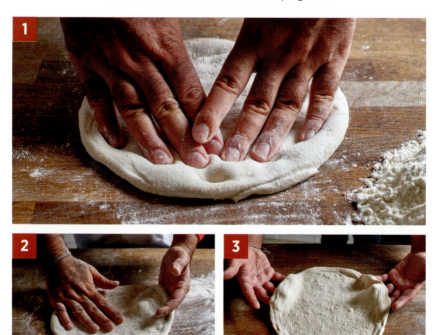

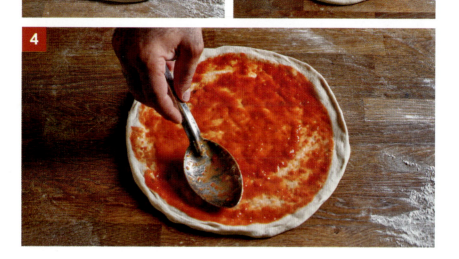

THE PIZZA DIET

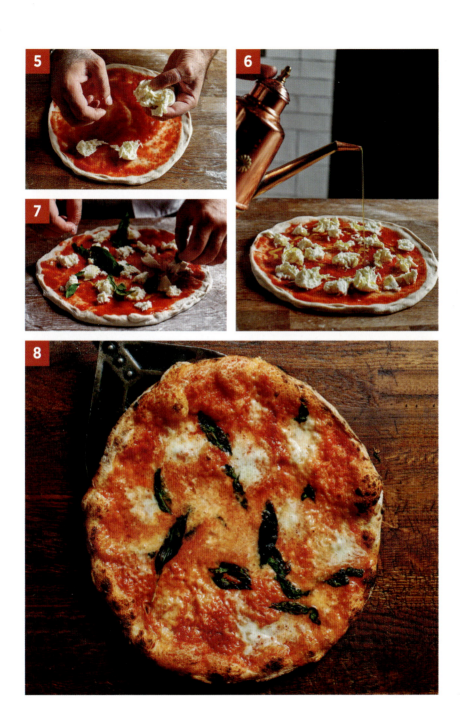

How to Bake Weight-Loss Pizzas

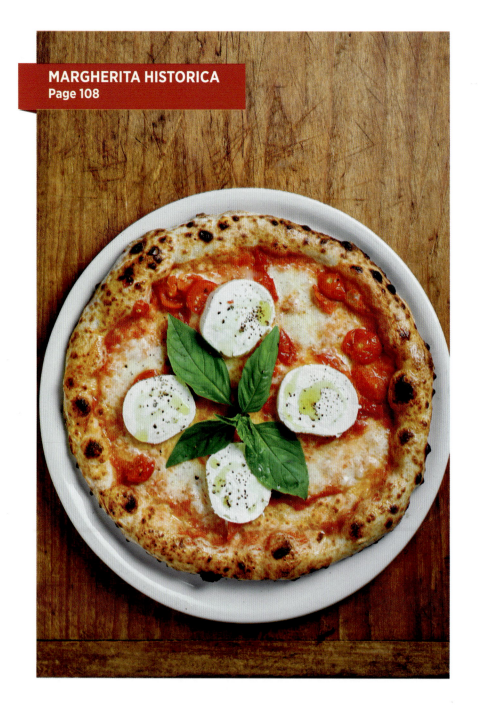

MARGHERITA HISTORICA
Page 108

THE PIZZA DIET

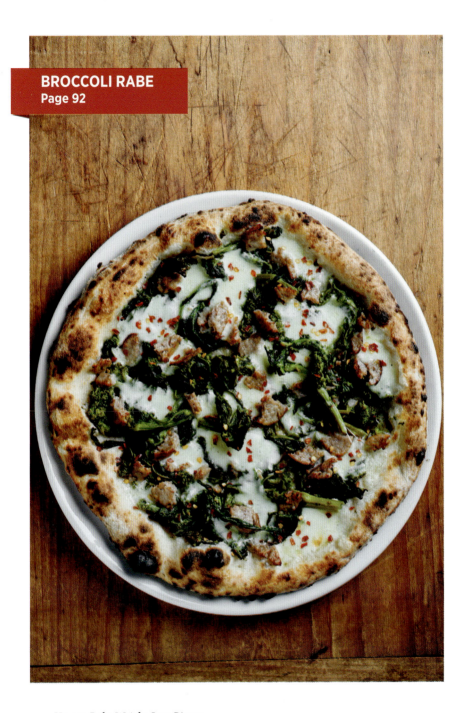

BROCCOLI RABE
Page 92

How to Bake Weight-Loss Pizzas

GRILLED VEGETABLE
Page 103

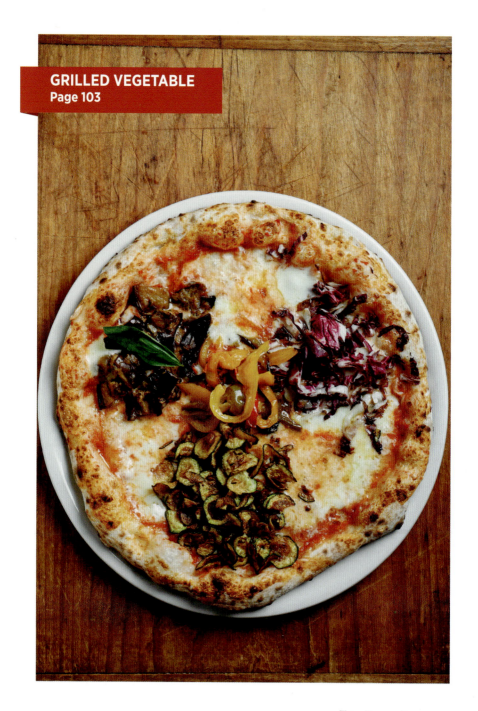

THE PIZZA DIET

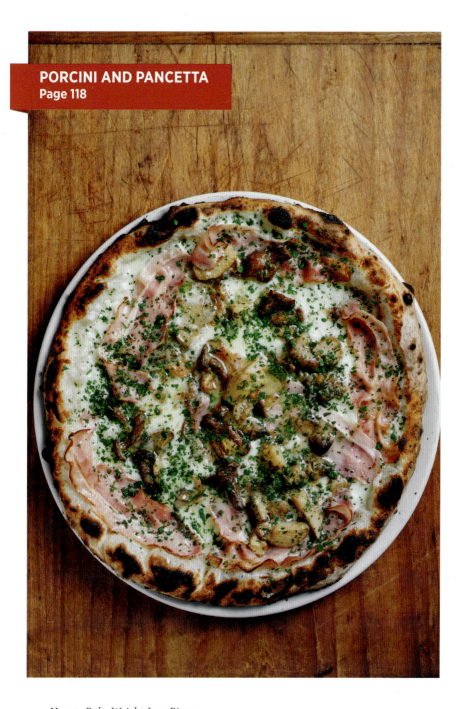

PORCINI AND PANCETTA
Page 118

How to Bake Weight-Loss Pizzas

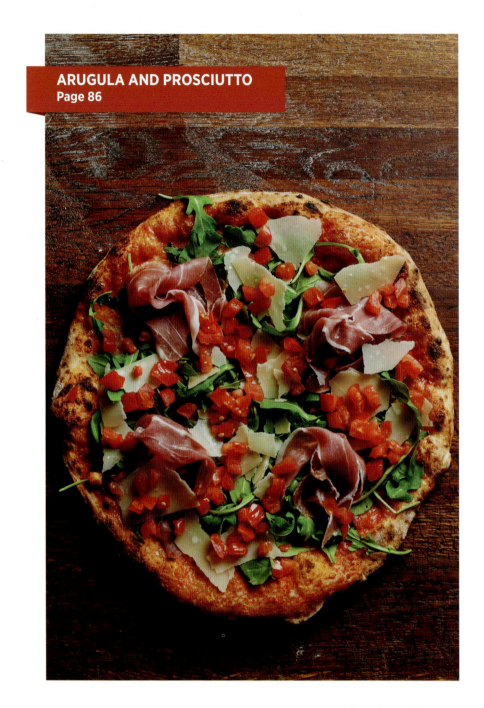

CAPRICCIOSA

3 Tbsp tomato sauce

8 oz pizza dough

1½ Tbsp chopped ham

2 canned artichokes packed in water, chopped

1 oz mushrooms, sliced

4 large basil leaves

6 black olives, sliced

2 oz fresh mozzarella, cubed

1 Tbsp extra-virgin olive oil

Preheat the oven to 500°F.

Place the pizza stone inside, if using.

Spread the tomato sauce on the dough. Top with the ham, artichokes, mushrooms, basil, olives and mozzarella.

Drizzle with olive oil. Bake on a parchment-lined baking sheet or a pizza stone for 10 to 11 minutes until the crust is golden brown.

CAULIFLOWER

1 Tbsp chicken or vegetable bouillon

½ head of cauliflower, cut into florets

2 Tbsp extra-virgin olive oil, divided

1 clove garlic, minced

8 oz pizza dough

2 oz fresh mozzarella, cubed

2 tsp fresh chopped parsley

Preheat the oven to 500°F.

Place the pizza stone inside, if using.

Bring 3 cups water to boil and add the bouillon. Boil the cauliflower for 5 to 6 minutes until soft. Drain. Heat a sauté pan with 1 tablespoon of olive oil over medium heat. Add the garlic and cauliflower and cook for 3 to 4 minutes. Remove from the heat and allow to cool.

Place the cauliflower mixture in a food processor and pulse until creamy. Spread the puree atop the dough, then add the cheese and parsley. Season with salt and pepper. Drizzle with 1 tablespoon olive oil.

Bake on a parchment-lined baking sheet or a pizza stone for 10 to 11 minutes until the crust is golden brown.

CHICKEN AND BELL PEPPER

2 tsp olive oil

7 oz chicken breast, cubed

2 Tbsp tomato sauce

8 oz pizza dough

1 red bell pepper, sliced

1 yellow bell pepper, sliced

2 oz fresh mozzarella, cubed

Preheat the oven to 500°F.

Place the pizza stone inside, if using.

Heat 1 teaspoon of olive oil in a pan over medium and cook the chicken about 4 minutes. Remove from heat and allow to cool.

Spread the tomato sauce on the dough. Top with the chicken, peppers, and mozzarella. Drizzle with 1 teaspoon olive oil. Season with salt and pepper.

Bake on a parchment-lined baking sheet or a pizza stone for 15 mintues until golden brown.

CLAM

7 oz fresh clams, such as Manila

1 Tbsp extra-virgin olive oil

1 Tbsp chopped white or yellow onion

5 Tbsp tomato sauce

2 tsp fresh chopped parsley

8 oz pizza dough

Preheat the oven to 500°F.

Place the pizza stone inside, if using.

Clean the clams well, brushing them and draining.

Heat a sauté pan over medium heat and add the clams. Cover and cook until the shells open. Remove from the pan and set aside.

Heat the olive oil and cook the onion until softened. Add the tomato sauce and season with salt and pepper. Cook until the water has evaporated, about 6 minutes. Remove from the heat, add the parsley and a little more olive oil and place in the refrigerator to cool.

Spread the tomato mixture atop the dough. Bake on a parchment-lined baking sheet or a pizza stone for 5 minutes.

Remove the clams from their shells and add to the pizza. Cook an additional 6 minutes until the crust is golden brown.

CRABMEAT

8 oz pizza dough

3 Tbsp fresh crabmeat

Pinch of chile flakes, to taste

½ onion, thinly sliced

2 oz fresh mozzarella, cubed

2 cups arugula, or as much as desired

1 Tbsp olive oil

Preheat the oven to 500°F.

Place the pizza stone inside, if using.

Top the dough with the crab, chile flakes, onion and mozzarella.

Bake on a parchment-lined baking sheet or a pizza stone for 14 minutes until golden brown.

Remove from the oven and top with the arugula. Season with a pinch of salt and a drizzle of olive oil.

Eat pizza the Italian way

In Italy, you get your own pizza, about the size of a dinner plate. If you don't want to look like a New York tourist, don't cut a slice and fold it. Use your knife and fork to cut bite-size pieces.

ESCAROLE AND CANNELLINI BEAN

7 oz cannellini beans, dried or canned

2 cloves garlic, minced

2 Tbsp + 1 tsp extra-virgin olive oil

1 bunch escarole

1 tsp chile flakes

8 oz pizza dough

Preheat the oven to 500°F.

Place the pizza stone inside, if using.

If using dried beans, soak them overnight. Then boil them for 25 to 30 minutes until soft. Five minutes before the beans are done, add a pinch of salt, half the garlic and 1 teaspoon olive oil. If using canned beans, drain them and rinse.

Rinse and dry the escarole. Heat 1 tablespoon olive oil over medium heat and add the other half of the garlic, the chile flakes and the escarole. Sauté until wilted and shiny, about 10 minutes. Stir in the beans and cook for another 10 minutes.

Drizzle the dough with 1 tablespoon olive oil and lightly dampen by dipping your fingers into a glass of water and flicking the water over top of the dough.

Bake on a parchment-lined baking sheet or a pizza stone for 6 minutes. Remove from the oven and spread the escarole-bean mixture on top.

Bake for an additional 4 minutes until the crust is golden brown.

GRILLED VEGETABLE

½ cup eggplant, sliced

½ cup zucchini, sliced

½ cup radiccio, chopped

½ bell pepper, sliced

2 Tbsp tomato sauce

8 oz pizza dough

2 oz fresh mozzarella, cubed

1 Tbsp extra-virgin olive oil

Preheat the oven to 500°F.

Place the pizza stone inside, if using.

Cook the vegetables on a grill or in a dry grill pan (without oil) over medium heat until softened and blackened on the edges, about 7 minutes. Sprinkle with sea salt. Let cool.

Spread the tomato sauce on the dough. Top with the mozzarella and then the grilled veggies. Drizzle with olive oil.

Bake on a parchment-lined baking sheet or a pizza stone for 10 to 11 minutes until the crust is golden brown.

GRILLED ZUCCHINI

1 zucchini, sliced into strips

8 oz pizza dough

2 oz fresh mozzarella, cubed

1 Tbsp extra-virgin olive oil

2 tsp fresh chopped parsley

Preheat the oven to 500°F.

Place the pizza stone inside, if using.

Cook the zucchini on a grill or in a grill pan until softened and blackened in spots, about 7 minutes. Remove from the heat and allow to cool.

Top the dough with the zucchini and mozzarella. Drizzle with olive oil. Bake on a parchment-lined baking sheet or a pizza stone for 12 minutes until the crust is golden brown.

Remove from the oven and sprinkle with parsley.

GUACAMOLE

1 avocado

Juice from half a lime

¼ tsp sea salt

½ red onion, diced

1 Tbsp chopped fresh cilantro

1 plum tomato, diced

1 small jalapeño, deseeded and diced (optional)

8 oz pizza dough

2 oz fresh mozzarella, cubed

1 Tbsp extra-virgin olive oil

Preheat the oven to 500°F.

Place the pizza stone inside, if using.

Prepare the guacamole. (Can also use high-quality store-bought.) Peel the avocado and mash in a bowl until slightly chunky. Mix with the lime juice and salt. Add the onion, cilantro, tomato and jalapeño (if using).

Top the dough with the mozzarella. Drizzle with olive oil. Bake on a parchment-lined baking sheet or a pizza stone for 12 minutes until the crust is golden brown.

Remove from the oven and spread the guacamole on top.

LOBSTER

8 oz pizza dough

1 small lobster tail

5 cherry tomatoes, quartered

1 tsp fresh grated ginger

1 shallot or 3 ramps, minced

2 oz fresh mozzarella, diced

1 Tbsp extra-virgin olive oil

Preheat the oven to 500°F.

Place the pizza stone inside, if using.

Bake the dough on a parchment-lined baking sheet or a pizza stone for 11 minutes until golden brown.

Bring an inch of salted water in a pot to boil. Place the lobster tail on a steamer rack and cover the pot. Cook for 8 minutes. Remove the lobster and allow to cool.

Remove the meat from the tail and chop. Mix with the cherry tomatoes, ginger, shallots, mozzarella and olive oil. Top the crust with the mixture.

MARGHERITA

3 Tbsp tomato sauce

8 oz pizza dough

4 large basil leaves

2 oz fresh mozzarella, cubed

1 Tbsp extra-virgin olive oil

Preheat the oven to 500°F.

Place the pizza stone inside, if using.

Spread the tomato sauce on the dough.

Top with the basil followed by the mozzarella cubes, evenly spaced across the pizza.

Drizzle with olive oil. Bake on a parchment-lined baking sheet or a pizza stone for 10 to 11 minutes until the crust is golden brown.

Always use fresh, local mozzarella

Never settle for the shredded mozzarella cheese that comes in a bag. It's loaded with preservatives and other junk, even wood pulp. You can do much better at a local cheese shop.

MARGHERITA HISTORICA

3 Tbsp tomato sauce

8 oz pizza dough

2 oz fresh buffalo mozzarella

4 large basil leaves

1 Tbsp extra-virgin olive oil

Preheat the oven to 500°F.

Place the pizza stone inside, if using.

Spread the tomato sauce on the dough. Top with the mozzarella and basil. Drizzle with olive oil.

Bake on a parchment-lined baking sheet or a pizza stone for 10 to 11 minutes until the crust is golden brown.

MARINARA

5 Tbsp tomato sauce

8 oz pizza dough

4 large basil leaves

1 clove garlic, sliced

1 tsp dried oregano

1 Tbsp extra-virgin olive oil

Preheat the oven to 500°F.

Place the pizza stone inside, if using.

Spread the tomato sauce on the dough.

Top with the basil, garlic and oregano. Drizzle with olive oil.

Bake on a parchment-lined baking sheet or a pizza stone for 10 to 11 minutes until the crust is golden brown.

Protect your brain with tomato sauce

Tomato-based foods like pizza are rich in lycopene, an antioxidant that can reduce your risk for stroke in part by lowering cholesterol and preventing blood clots, according to a study in the journal *Neurology*.

How to Cool a Pizza Burn

If you eat enough pizza, you're bound to get burned. Who hasn't bitten into a piping hot slice and singed their tongue or the roof of their mouth with bubbling cheese?

The best home remedies involve cooling the burn as soon as it happens:

▶ **Drink ice water** to reduce the heat and inflammation on the thin tissue of your tongue or roof of your mouth.

▶ **Put an ice cube** in your mouth directly on the burn to bring down the temperature and swelling, which will ease the pain.

▶ **Spoonfuls of cool yogurt or ice cream** will help cool and soothe the burn.

▶ **Countless grandmothers** swear by this old home remedy: White sugar crystals spread on the angry parts of your mouth.

MARINARA WITH SARDINES

2 Tbsp tomato sauce

8 oz pizza dough

2 oz boneless sardines, canned or fresh, chopped

4 cherry tomatoes, quartered

1 tsp dried oregano

2 tsp fresh chopped parsley

1 tsp extra-virgin olive oil

Preheat the oven to 500°F.

Place the pizza stone inside, if using.

Spread the tomato sauce on the dough. Add the sardines, tomatoes, oregano, parsley, and olive oil.

Bake on a parchment-lined baking sheet or a pizza stone for 14 minutes until golden brown.

MUSHROOM

4 oz cremini, portobello or shiitake mushrooms, sliced

1 Tbsp extra-virgin olive oil

1 clove garlic, minced

2 tsp fresh chopped parsley

3 Tbsp tomato sauce

8 oz pizza dough

2 oz fresh mozzarella, cubed

Preheat the oven to 500°F.

Place the pizza stone inside, if using.

Heat a dry sauté pan over medium heat. Add the mushrooms, season with a pinch of sea salt, cover and cook for 6 to 7 minutes, until the mushrooms have released their liquid. Drain and remove from the pan.

Add 1 tablespoon olive oil and the garlic to the pan. Sauté the mushrooms for 3 to 4 minutes until browned. Remove from the heat. Season with salt and pepper and sprinkle with parsley. Allow to cool.

Spread the tomato sauce on the dough. Top with the mushroom mixture and the mozzarella. Bake on a parchment-lined baking sheet or a pizza stone for 10 to 11 minutes until the crust is golden brown.

MUSSEL

8 oz pizza dough

6 Tbsp + 2 tsp tomato sauce

1 clove garlic, minced

1 Tbsp extra-virgin olive oil

10 fresh mussels

2 tsp fresh chopped parsley

Preheat the oven to 500°F.

Place the pizza stone inside, if using.

Top the dough with the tomato sauce and garlic. Season with pepper. Drizzle with 1 tablespoon olive oil.

Bake on a parchment-lined baking sheet or a pizza stone for 12 minutes until the crust is golden brown. Take the crust out of the oven.

Clean the mussels and then add atop the cooked pizza crust and bake for an additional 5 minutes. Sprinkle with the parsley before serving.

Mussels for brains

Farmed or wild, mussels are a great source of protein, omega-3s and vitamin B_{12}, a nutrient critical to proper brain and nervous system function.

OCTOPUS

8 oz pizza dough

2 oz tomato sauce

8 cherry tomatoes, quartered

5 capers

5 black olives, sliced

1 fresh baby octopus, roughly chopped

2 Tbsp chopped pistachios

1½ cups arugula

Preheat the oven to 500°F.

Place the pizza stone inside, if using.

Top the dough with the tomato sauce, tomatoes, capers and olives. Bake on a parchment-lined baking sheet or a pizza stone for 6 minutes.

Add the octopus and bake another 8 minutes or until the crust is golden brown. Remove and top with pistachios and arugula.

When the fire's hot, take your pizza for a spin

When cooking a pizza in a wood-fired oven, the side closest to the fire will char quickly unless you keep the pizza rotating. Chefs use a metal pallino for this instead of a wooden peel, deftly spinning the pie 90 degrees every 20 seconds.

ONION CALZONE

8 oz pizza dough

1 red onion, thinly sliced

1 Tbsp pecorino cheese, grated

2 tsp extra-virgin olive oil, divided

Preheat the oven to 500°F.

Place the pizza stone inside, if using.

Divide the dough ball into two equal parts and flatten to create two discs of equal size, roughly 6 inches across.

Place the onion in the middle of the first disc. Sprinkle with the cheese and drizzle with 1 teaspoon olive oil. Season with a pinch of sea salt.

Place the other disc on top of the first, and pinch-seal the two discs around the edges to create a packet. Brush the top with olive oil.

Bake on a parchment-lined baking sheet or a pizza stone for 15 minutes until the crust is golden brown.

OYSTERS GRATIN

5 oysters, fresh, such as Blue Point, in shell

1 Tbsp + 1 tsp bread crumbs

1 clove garlic, minced

2 tsp fresh chopped parsley

Chile flakes to taste

2 Tbsp extra-virgin olive oil, divided

8 oz pizza dough

3 Tbsp tomato sauce

Preheat the oven to 500°F.

Place the pizza stone inside, if using.

Open the oyster shells with a knife, discarding the top half of the shell. In a small bowl, combine the bread crumbs, garlic, parsley and chile flakes and top each oyster-in-the-half-shell with an equal amount of the mixture. Drizzle with olive oil.

Put onto a baking sheet and bake for 10 minutes in the top half of the oven.

Spread the dough with the tomato sauce. Drizzle with 1 tablespoon olive oil and bake for 10 minutes in the bottom half of the oven, as the oysters cook.

Place the oysters atop the dough and bake for an additional 3 to 5 minutes.

PEAR, WALNUT AND COTTAGE CHEESE

2 oz cottage cheese

8 oz pizza dough

1 pear, sliced

2 Tbsp chopped walnuts

1 Tbsp blue cheese

Preheat the oven to 500°F.

Place the pizza stone inside, if using.

Spread the cottage cheese across the dough. Top with the pear, walnuts and blue cheese. Season with salt and pepper.

Bake on a parchment-lined baking sheet or a pizza stone for 15 minutes until golden brown.

Dos and dough nots

Be careful to avoid making your dough so thin that you get holes. And remember that the thinner the dough, the more quickly it will cook—and burn.

PORCINI AND PANCETTA

4 oz porcini mushrooms

6 very thin slices fat-free Italian bacon or panchetta

2 oz fresh mozzarella, cubed

1 Tbsp extra-virgin olive oil

8 oz pizza dough

3 Tbsp tomato sauce

2 tsp fresh parsley, chopped

Sea salt, pinch

Preheat the oven to 500°F.

Place the pizza stone inside, if using.

Heat a dry sauté pan over medium heat. Add the mushrooms, season with a pinch of sea salt, cover and cook for 6 to 7 minutes, until the mushrooms have released their liquid. Drain and remove from the pan.

Top the dough with the tomato sauce, mozzarella, porcini mushrooms, slices of bacon, and parsley. Drizzle with 1 tablespoon olive oil.

Bake on a parchment-lined baking sheet or a pizza stone for 10 to 11 minutes or until the crust is golden brown.

PUMPKIN, SPINACH AND RICOTTA

1 bunch fresh spinach

2 Tbsp fresh ricotta cheese

1 egg

8 oz pizza dough

2 oz fresh mozzarella, cubed

1 small roasted pumpkin slice, chopped

Sprinkle of saffron

Chile flakes to taste

Preheat the oven to 500°F.

Place the pizza stone inside, if using.

Boil the spinach in salted water for 3 to 4 minutes. Drain and allow to cool. Place in a food processor with the ricotta and the egg. Pulse until blended.

Top the dough with the mozzarella, pumpkin and the saffron. Then spread on the spinach-ricotta mixture. Add a sprinkle of chile flakes, if desired.

Bake on a parchment-lined baking sheet or a pizza stone for 15 minutes until the crust is golden brown.

RAW MUSHROOM AND SPINACH

2 oz cremini mushrooms, thinly sliced

1 handful of baby spinach

2 tsp extra-virgin olive oil, divided

1 lemon wedge

8 oz pizza dough

2 oz goat cheese, crumbled

Preheat the oven to 500°F.

Place the pizza stone inside, if using.

Toss the mushrooms and spinach with 1 teaspoon olive oil and a squeeze of lemon juice. Season with salt and pepper.

Drizzle the dough with 1 teaspoon olive oil. Sprinkle with a pinch of sea salt.

Bake on a parchment-lined baking sheet or a pizza stone for 14 minutes until golden brown.

Remove from the oven and top with the mushroom-spinach salad and the goat cheese.

RICOTTA AND TOMATO CALZONE

2 oz fresh mozzarella, cubed

2 Tbsp fresh ricotta cheese

4 large basil leaves

8 oz pizza dough

1 tsp extra-virgin olive oil

1 Tbsp tomato sauce

Preheat the oven to 500°F.

Place the pizza stone inside, if using.

Place the mozzarella, ricotta and basil on one half of the dough.

Fold the dough over the filling to form a half-moon shape. Seal the edges with your fingers or a fork. Brush the top with a little oil and poke a hole to allow steam to escape.

Bake on a parchment-lined baking sheet or a pizza stone for 14 minutes until golden brown.

Remove from the oven and spread the tomato sauce across the top.

ROASTED PEPPER

1 bell pepper

2 tsp capers

5 black olives, sliced

1 Tbsp extra-virgin olive oil

8 oz pizza dough

2 oz fresh mozzarella, cubed

Preheat the oven to 500°F.

Place the pizza stone inside, if using.

Cook the pepper on a grill or in a grill pan for 10 minutes until blackened in spots. Remove from the heat, cool and cut into thin slices. Mix with the capers, olives and olive oil and spread on the dough. Add the mozzarella.

Bake on a parchment-lined baking sheet or a pizza stone for 10 to 11 minutes until the crust is golden brown.

SALAD PIZZA

8 oz pizza dough

1 Tbsp + 1 tsp extra-virgin olive oil

6 lettuce leaves

4 canned anchovy fillets, chopped

1 tsp capers

4 green olives, sliced

4 black olives, sliced

1 clove garlic, minced

Preheat the oven to 500°F.

Place the pizza stone inside, if using.

Drizzle the dough with 1 tablespoon olive oil. Bake on a parchment-lined baking sheet or a pizza stone for 10 to 11 minutes until the crust is golden brown.

Remove from the oven and arrange the lettuce leaves atop. Then place the anchovy fillets, capers, olives and garlic. Drizzle with the remaining olive oil and season with salt and a generous pinch of pepper.

SALMON AND MOZZARELLA

8 oz pizza dough

2 oz fresh mozzarella, cubed

3.5 oz smoked salmon, chopped

2 tsp fresh chopped parsley

Preheat the oven to 500°F.

Place the pizza stone inside, if using.

Top the dough with the mozzarella, salmon, parsley and a sprinkle of black pepper.

Bake on a parchment-lined baking sheet or a pizza stone for 10 to 11 minutes until the crust is golden brown.

(Alternatively, this pizza can be made with 3 tablespoons of tomato sauce. Simply top the dough with the sauce before adding the other ingredients.)

SCALLOP

¼ cup frozen green peas

¼ cup onion, thinly sliced

2 tsp extra-virgin olive oil, divided

4 fresh, medium scallops

8 oz pizza dough

1 Tbsp pecorino cheese, grated

2 tsp fresh chopped parsley

Preheat the oven to 500°F.

Place the pizza stone inside, if using.

Boil the peas in 1 cup water with a pinch of sea salt, the onion, and 1 teaspoon extra-virgin olive oil. When half the water has evaporated, remove from the heat and transfer the peas, onion and remaining water to a food processor. Blend to form a thick cream.

Heat a pan with 1 teaspoon olive oil over medium heat and sear the scallops, 2 minutes on each side. Remove from the heat and allow to cool.

Spread the pea mixture on the dough. Top with the scallops.

Bake on a parchment-lined baking sheet or a pizza stone for 10 to 11 minutes until the crust is golden brown.

Remove from the oven and sprinkle with pecorino cheese and parsley.

SHRIMP

5 fresh shrimp, heads removed

3 stalks asparagus

8 oz pizza dough

1 Tbsp extra-virgin olive oil

2 oz smoked mozzarella, cubed

Preheat the oven to 500°F.

Place the pizza stone inside, if using.

Bring an inch of salted water in a pot to boil. Place the shrimp and asparagus on a steamer rack and cover the pot. Cook for 5 minutes. Remove from the heat and allow to cool. Discard the shrimp shells and tails. Cut the asparagus in half lengthwise.

Drizzle the dough with olive oil and top with the mozzarella. Bake on a parchment-lined baking sheet or a pizza stone for 6 minutes.

Top with the asparagus and shrimp and bake for an additional 6 minutes.

SLICED BEEF

2 tsp extra-virgin olive oil, divided

2 oz veal, cut into strips

2 lemon wedges

8 oz pizza dough

2 cups arugula, or as much as desired

4 slices of shaved Parmesan cheese

Preheat the oven to 500°F.

Place the pizza stone inside, if using.

Heat a pan with 1 teaspoon olive oil over medium heat. Add the veal. Season with salt and pepper and cook for 3 minutes. Remove from the heat and dress with a squeeze of lemon juice.

Drizzle 1 teaspoon olive oil on the dough. Season with a sprinkle of sea salt.

Bake on a parchment-lined baking sheet or a pizza stone for 14 minutes until golden brown.

Remove from the oven and top with arugula, veal, and Parmesan. Dress with a squeeze of lemon.

SPINACH

1 bunch fresh spinach

2 Tbsp ricotta cheese

8 oz pizza dough

2 oz fresh mozzarella, cubed

2 tsp fresh rosemary

5 cherry tomatoes, quartered

1 handful of mixed greens, including lettuce, endive and arugula

Preheat the oven to 500°F.

Place the pizza stone inside, if using.

Rinse the spinach and boil in salted water for 3 minutes.

Drain and let cool. Place in a food processor with the ricotta and a pinch of sea salt. Blend until creamy.

Smear the spinach cream atop the dough.

Bake on a parchment-lined baking sheet or a pizza stone for 10 to 11 minutes.

Remove from the oven, add the mozzarella and bake for an additional 5 minutes until the cheese is melted.

Remove from the oven and top with rosemary, tomatoes and greens.

SPINACH AND RICOTTA

2 oz ricotta cheese

8 oz pizza dough

3.5 oz fresh spinach

2 oz ham, cubed

Preheat the oven to 500°F.

Place the pizza stone inside, if using.

Spread the ricotta atop the dough. Then add a layer of spinach and finish with the ham.

Bake on a parchment-lined baking sheet or a pizza stone for 10 to 11 minutes until the crust is golden brown.

Tame your hunger with a topping of greens

Spinach can stifle hunger and cravings thanks to compounds in the vegetable's cells that promote the release of satiety hormones.

SULTANA

2 tsp raisins

2 Tbsp extra-virgin olive oil, divided

4 leaves of escarole or white endive

.7 oz pitted black olives

1 handful of capers

1 canned anchovy fillet, chopped

8 oz pizza dough

1 handful of pine nuts

Preheat the oven to 500°F.

Place the pizza stone inside, if using.

Soak the raisins in warm water for 15 minutes. Drain.

Heat 1 tablespoon olive oil in a pan over medium heat and sauté the escarole (or endive) with the olives, capers and anchovy, about 10 minutes. Remove from the heat and let cool.

Brush the dough with olive oil and top with the escarole mixture. Add the pine nuts and raisins. Drizzle with 1 tablespoon olive oil.

Bake on a parchment-lined baking sheet or a pizza stone for 12 minutes until the crust is golden brown.

TOMATO AND ROCKET

8 oz pizza dough

2 oz smoked mozzarella, cubed

8 cherry tomatoes, quartered

1 Tbsp extra-virgin olive oil

2 cups arugula

4 very thin slices of prosciutto di Parma

Preheat the oven to 450°F.

Place the pizza stone inside, if using.

Top the dough with the mozzarella and cherry tomatoes. Drizzle with olive oil.

Bake on a parchment-lined baking sheet or a pizza stone for 10 to 11 minutes until the crust is golden brown.

Remove from the oven and top with arugula and the prosciutto di Parma.

Indeed it is rocket science!

"Rocket" is another, very European, word for arugula, the salad leaf with the peppery bite. You might see it as "rucola" on a menu. Same thing. It's low-cal and very high in folate, sulforaphane and other healthy nutrients.

TUNA

8 oz pizza dough

3 Tbsp tomato sauce

2 oz fresh mozzarella, cubed

1 stalk celery, diced

1 small onion, minced

5 capers

5 black olives, sliced

2 oz canned tuna in oil, crumbled

1 Tbsp extra-virgin olive oil

Preheat the oven to 500°F.

Place the pizza stone inside, if using.

Top the dough with the tomato sauce and mozzarella. Add the celery, onion, capers, olives, and tuna. Drizzle with olive oil. Bake on a parchment-lined baking sheet or a pizza stone for 10 to 11 minutes until the crust is golden brown.

A tuna helper

Topping your pizza with canned tuna is a quick way to add protein and omega-3s to your meal. It's inexpensive and ready in seconds if it's in your pantry.

VEGAN

Seasonal grilled vegetables, including eggplant, pepper and zucchini, sliced

8 oz pizza dough

2 oz firm tofu, diced

1 Tbsp extra-virgin olive oil

Preheat the oven to 500°F.

Place the pizza stone inside, if using.

Cook the vegetable slices on a grill or in a grill pan for 7 minutes until softened and blackened in spots.

Bake the dough on a parchment-lined baking sheet or a pizza stone for 14 minutes until golden brown.

Remove from the oven and add the grilled vegetables and tofu. Season with sea salt and a drizzle of olive oil.

Spread the tomato sauce on the dough. Top with the chicken, peppers, and mozzarella. Drizzle with 1 teaspoon olive oil. Season with salt and pepper.

Bake on a parchment-lined baking sheet or a pizza stone for 15 mintues until golden brown.

ZUCCHINI BLOSSOM

8 oz pizza dough

5 zucchini blossoms

4 canned anchovy fillets, chopped

2 oz fresh mozzarella, cubed

1 Tbsp extra-virgin olive oil

Preheat the oven to 500°F.

Place the pizza stone inside, if using.

Top the dough with the zucchini blossoms, anchovies, and mozzarella. Drizzle with olive oil.

Bake on a parchment-lined baking sheet or a pizza stone for 14 minutes until golden brown.

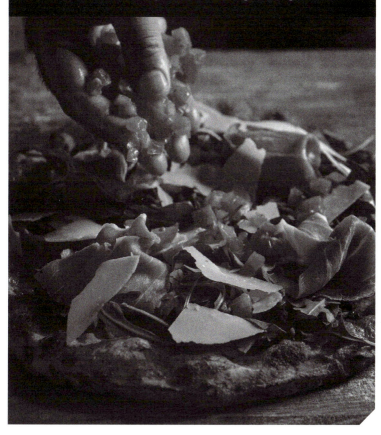

Chapter 7

Top Your Pizza with Superfoods

A shopping guide to the toppings that'll upgrade the nutritional profile of your pizza

135

I love the classic, simple cheese pizza where the mozzarella and sauce, some fragrant basil and, of course, a crispy crust combine their unique textures and flavors to create one of the most delicious meals you'll ever eat.

Simplicity goes a long way in the culinary arts. But if you're eating a pizza for lunch every day, as I do, you'll want a change of taste now and then. Toppings bring versatility of flavor to your pizza, and there's unlimited opportunity for creativity by combining them just so.

Pizza toppings also can make your pizza more nutritious and healthful by adding extra vitamins, minerals, and fiber. Pizza toppings also can be calorie bombs, especially the fatty meat toppings like sausage, pepperoni, and meatballs. So you need to practice mindful eating even while enjoying your midday treat.

I'm not a nutritionist by any means, I'm a chef from Naples, but fortunately my partners, the editors at *Eat This, Not That!* magazine, are experts at gathering healthy-living information and have supplied me with the latest nutrition and weight-loss research. Try these favorite and exotic toppings alone or in combination on your pizzas. They'll add a level of flavor and nutrition that will help you get the most out of the Pizza Diet.

THE PIZZA DIET TOPPINGS

ANCHOVIES

Just two slices of anchovy pizza will get you more than halfway to your daily quota of heart-healthy omega-3 fatty acids. Anchovies also are rich in calcium and potassium (both essential weight-loss minerals) as well as vitamin A. The downside of anchovies on your pizza is the added salt. If you want to reduce sodium but still want fish on your pizza, try sardines, which are much less salty and deliver more protein.

ARTICHOKES

This fiber-rich plant contains more bone-building magnesium and potassium than any other vegetable. The leaves contain antioxidants that can reduce stroke risk and vitamin C for immune-system health.

ARUGULA

Arugula is a tangy, peppery leafy green that provides as many nutritional health benefits as better-known kale and Brussels sprouts. A key nutrient in arugula is alpha-lipoic acid, which is used to reverse hardening of the blood vessels and prevent heart attacks and also lowers blood sugar. Like other cruciferous vegetables, it contains a powerful cancer-fighting nutrient called sulforaphane, plus calcium and vitamin K. While arugula looks beautiful atop a pizza pie, it can also be hidden inside if you cook it with your sauce, a trick that can help you get your kids to eat more vegetables.

BASIL

Fresh basil is an aromatic herb that coaxes out the natural sweetness of the tomatoes without overpowering the flavor of the sauce or the cheese. Delicate, but powerful, basil leaves and stems contain essential oils and phytochemicals that have biological activity in the body, especially as an anti-inflammatory. Basil essential oils have been shown to lower blood glucose and triglyceride and cholesterol levels. And there is nothing better to top leftover pizza with the next day that will make the pie taste fresh baked.

BELL PEPPERS

Topping your pizza with sliced bell peppers can be an easy way to lower your cholesterol while adding texture and flavor to your pie. A study conducted at the University of Michigan, Ann Arbor, reveals that beta-carotene-rich foods, like bell peppers, can increase the proportion of beneficial HDL cholesterol to total cholesterol in rats, potentially reducing the risk of stroke and heart disease in those with high cholesterol. Tip: You'll enjoy peppers even more on your pie if you roast them first.

BROCCOLI (and broccolini)

This cruciferous vegetable is loaded with the potent nutrient sulforaphane, which has powerful anticancer properties, according to studies at Johns Hopkins University. Other good sources of the phytonutrient are cauliflower, Brussels sprouts, and kale. Try some on your next pie.

EGGPLANT

Eggplant is good for more than just parmigiana. Thin slices of the shiny, purple vegetable make a nice, nutritious pizza topping as a meat replacement. It's packed with powerful antioxidants called anthocyanins that provide neuroprotective benefits like boosting short-term memory and reducing inflammation.

FLAXSEEDS

This may sound nuts, but these tiny seeds are packed with fiber, vitamin B_1, magnesium and heart-healthy omega-3s. Add a tablespoon to your sauce or sprinkle on top of the cheese after the pizza has baked. You'll hardly taste it, and it adds only 35 calories.

GARLIC

Keep the powdered stuff on the shelf. Roasted garlic adds a mellow yet still pungent note to the flavor profile of your pie. Also try fresh garlic sliced thin, chopped, crushed or minced. It's good for your cardiovascular system, keeping blood vessels flexible as you age. And it contains strong antibacterial powers.

HOT PEPPERS

Capsaicin, the chemical that gives hot peppers their bite, may raise your metabolism to burn more calories and help you lose weight, according to some studies. Other research in the journal *Open Heart* reveals that the capsaicin found in hot peppers can lower cholesterol.

KALE

Like almonds, kale kind of started the whole superfood obsession. It's a hearty green, meaning it takes a little more getting used to than other greens like spinach, but it's worth it. Kale is rich in phytochemicals like lutein and zeaxanthin that help maintain eyesight. It also contains a bunch of vital nutrients like phosphorus, vitamin E and folate.

MEATBALLS AND OTHER MEATS

For the most part, topping a pizza with meat, especially meatballs, pepperoni or bacon, will overpower the flavor of the cheese and sauce and leave greasy fat that you don't need when trying to lose weight. If you want to load up on protein, add slices of lean chicken breast or anchovies/sardines (see above). If you must have processed meats, keep them to a minimum and only on occasion. Remember, the key principle of the Pizza Diet is learning to be mindful of what you are eating. By being careful in your choices, you can lose weight quickly and easily without feeling as if you are sacrificing your favorite foods.

MUSHROOMS

They're a common pizza topping, but why be common? Sample the nuanced flavors of shiitake, maitake, reishi and portobello mushrooms and others. All mushrooms contain significant cholesterol- and cancer-fighting properties. They are rich in potassium, which helps the heart maintain normal rhythm, fluid balance and nerve function, and selenium. A recent study published in the *British Journal of Urology* found that men who eat plenty of selenium-rich foods can reduce their risk of prostate cancer.

ONIONS

If you have high cholesterol, the only tears you should be shedding while chopping onions for your pizza are tears of joy. Researchers from the University of Colorado at Boulder's Department of Evolutionary Biology found that antioxidant-rich onions can help those who consume them maintain a healthier LDL-to-HDL ratio.

PINEAPPLE

You will never find this on a pizza in Napoli, but if you like sweet, juicy fruit on your pie, this one contains a potent mix of vitamins and enzymes that lower inflammation and have been shown to protect against arthritis and macular degeneration.

ROMA TOMATOES

One reason pizza is considered health food is because cooked tomatoes and tomato paste deliver even more of the heart-healthy nutrient lycopene than fresh ones do. But don't discount slicing some fresh meaty Romas as a topping. More lycopene is always better. It has been shown to protect against degenerative brain diseases and prostate cancer.

SPINACH

This fairly common topping is an excellent source of vitamins and minerals, calcium, fiber and protein, and is also very low in calories. And due to its subtle flavor and texture, spinach on your pizza boosts the nutritional value of every bite without overpowering the other flavors. (Try it in combination with artichoke hearts.) You might not even notice you ate spinach pizza, until you look in the mirror and see it on your teeth.

SUN-DRIED TOMATOES

Just 1 cup of sun-dried tomatoes delivers you 7 grams of fiber, three-quarters of your recommended daily allowance (RDA) of potassium—which is essential for heart health and tissue repair—and 50 percent of your RDA of vitamin C, the superstar antioxidant that prevents DNA damage. They're also rich in vitamins A and K, and metabolism-revving potassium.

SWEET POTATOES

Yes, sweet potatoes. Slice them thin like large rings of pepperoni. They are better for you than the popular pizza topping. Sweet potatoes contain glutathione, an antioxidant that boosts immune-system health and may protect against Alzheimer's and Parkinson's diseases, heart attack, stroke and diabetes.

WATERCRESS

This leafy green made headlines when it topped the list of powerhouse foods in a study conducted by researchers at William Paterson University in New Jersey, which measured the nutritional density of various foods. Watercress surprised everyone by significantly outranking kale in the results. Consuming this superfood has been credited with helping to lower blood pressure, cutting your risk for cancer and diabetes and helping to keep bones healthy. Watercress is often used in salads, but its peppery flavor works well on top of pizza. But don't go overboard; a little goes a long way.

Chapter 8

What to Eat When Not Eating Pizza

Strategies and recipes to help you embrace the foods of the Mediterranean lifestyle

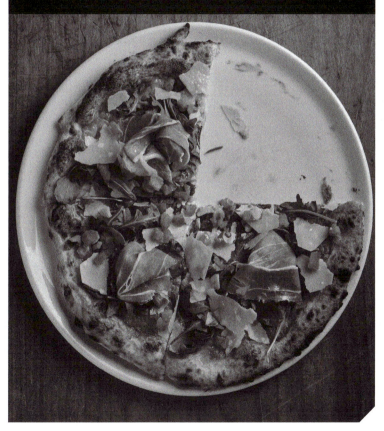

Whether you eat your pizza for breakfast (Italy has witnessed an 8 percent increase in people eating pizza for breakfast over recent years), lunch or dinner doesn't really matter. What matters is that when you aren't eating your homemade pizza you are eating a Mediterranean-style diet, which means you're eating modestly from a wide variety of fresh, whole foods, mostly plants. I'm going to assume that you're having your pizza for lunch. That means you need some direction for breakfast and dinner. It's simple, really.

Just make sure your bowl or plate contains this:

▶ **PROTEIN • FIBER • HEALTHY FATS**

And not that:

▶ **HIGHLY PROCESSED CARBOHYDRATES**

Here's how to make the the Pizza Diet easy for you.

BREAKFAST

A lot of people call it the most crucial meal of the day. The jury is still out on just how crucial it is to weight loss. Some studies have shown that those who skip breakfast tend to gain more weight than those who don't. For some people, fasting for 16 hours, from just after dinner at 7 p.m. until noon the next day, is an effective way to lose weight.

For me, I always eat breakfast, and I recommend you do, too, for one important reason: You'll feel fuller as the day drags on, making you less likely to reach for unhealthy snacks or to binge-eat an entire buffet for lunch.

Our appetite is regulated by hormones. One called ghrelin tells our brain we're hungry and screams, "Get yourself to a

McDonald's." Another hormone called leptin sends a signal to our brain when we're full, telling our hands to stop shoveling food down our throat. The problem is, when we diet, our ghrelin levels spike, making us hungrier. And as we gain more weight, our bodies produce less leptin, making it harder to tell when we're full and requiring us to eat even more before we're satisfied.

It's a vicious cycle that's best avoided.

The key, I've found, is to retrain your body to feel satiated, and I learned how to do it, in part, by eating the right kinds of food at breakfast. You have to choose foods that are nutritious, that contain slow-burning proteins, complex carbohydrates and fiber, and keep you filled up.

Sugars and processed carbs (such as anything made with white flour) that give you a quick spike in energy but leave you hungry again soon enough should be avoided.

Fruits are a better choice. They're packed with fiber, which helps send that "full" signal to your brain. Try sprinkling your cereal with blueberries or sliced strawberries, or eat a whole apple.

As I mentioned earlier, protein is the most satisfying of the food groups. Nuts are a solid plant-based source, especially almonds, which are relatively low in calories and full of protein. I often top my cereal with sliced almonds and eat it with home-made almond milk.

And speaking of cereal, it's what I eat for breakfast more than anything else. It's quick, and I sometimes don't have a lot of time in the morning, as I try to wrestle my young son into whatever outfit he's picked to wear to school. But most cereals are overly processed, full of sugar and pretty much devoid of nutrition. (Hint: If there's a toy inside the box, you shouldn't be eating it.)

What to Eat When Not Eating Pizza

You can, however, make a healthy choice, even with boxed cereals. Choose ones whose ingredients are as close to their original form as possible. If it says it contains almonds, you should see something that looks like actual almonds in your bowl. Also spend a little time with the ingredient and nutrition label. The cereal should be loaded with whole grains, such as oats, shredded wheat or barley. The sugar content should be low—under 10 grams per serving. Less, if possible. Grape-Nuts, for example, only has 5 grams in a ½-cup serving. Make sure your cereal has also got belly-filling fiber—at least 3 grams.

My friends at *Eat This, Not That!* magazine and EatThis.com analyze and critique groceries and restaurant foods all the time. Recently, they recommended some excellent high-fiber breakfast cereals without added sugars. Try these out with a topping of berries for sweetness:

Quaker Instant Oatmeal Original
Bob's Red Mill Gluten-Free Classic Oatmeal with Flax and Chia
Post Shredded Wheat, Wheat 'n' Bran
General Mills Fiber One
McCann's Quick-Cooking Rolled Oats Irish Oatmeal
Ezekiel 4:9 Almond Sprouted-Grain Crunchy Cereal
Barbara's Shredded Wheat

Here are a few ideas for quick, filling and nutritious morning meals, followed by some more detailed breakfast recipes for when you have more time to cook. Mix and match all week.

Make your own almond milk. It's easy to do, and you'll know it'll be free of the preservatives and thickeners some store-bought varieties contain. Try this recipe: Combine 2 ounces organic blanched almonds with ⅔ cup warm water in a blender. Blend until smooth. Strain through a cheesecloth into a glass bottle or airtight container and add a pinch of sea salt. Store in the refrigerator for up to 3 days.

Top ½ cup cereal with ¼ cup almond milk. Sprinkle on a small handful of sliced almonds, blueberries or sliced strawberries. Feel free to pair your cereal with a cup of black coffee, sweetened with 1 teaspoon of pure maple syrup. Or have a mug of green tea with a splash of almond milk.

For a heartier breakfast, have one sunny-side-up egg with a side of dry whole-wheat toast and an apple. Wash it down with black coffee or espresso and a tall glass of water.

Have one slice of whole-wheat toast spread with fruit preserves. (Look for brands that are all natural and made without high-fructose corn syrup.) Pair with a skim milk cappuccino.

Make one 3-inch gluten-free pancake. I use a boxed mix from Trader Joe's, which is made with rice flour—a better source of fiber and protein than plain old white flour. Top your pancake with 1 teaspoon pure maple syrup and 1 teaspoon unsalted Irish butter.

Blend a breakfast smoothie. Try these three recipes.

1. Cherry-Banana: Combine ½ cup cherries, ½ frozen banana, ¼ lime, ¼ cup unsweetened almond milk, 1 scoop plant-based plain protein powder, and 3 ice cubes. Blend on high until smooth.

2. Banana-Mango: Combine 1 ripe banana, ¾ cup frozen mango pieces, ½ cup orange juice, ¼ cup Greek yogurt. If the smoothie is too thick, add a few splashes of water and blend again.

3. **Banana Joe:** 1 very ripe banana, ½ cup strong coffee, ½ cup milk, 1 Tbsp peanut butter, 1 Tbsp agave syrup, 1 cup ice. Blend.

BACON, LETTUCE, TOMATO, AND EGG SANDWICH

1 egg

2 slices 7-grain or sourdough bread, lightly toasted

Handful of arugula

3 thick slices tomato

4 strips bacon, cooked

Salt and black pepper to taste

Heat a small nonstick skillet over medium heat. Coat with olive oil cooking spray and add the egg. Cook sunny side up until the white is set but the yolk is runny.

Line the bottom half of the bread with the arugula, followed by the tomato slices and bacon. Set the cooked egg carefully on top and season with a pinch of salt and plenty of fresh cracked pepper. Top with the second slice of bread. Makes one serving.

BAKED EGG WITH MUSHROOMS AND SPINACH

1 Tbsp olive oil

1 small onion, chopped

2 cups mushrooms, sliced

4 slices Canadian bacon or deli ham, cut into thin strips

½ (10 oz) bag frozen spinach, thawed

½ (7 oz) can roasted green chiles

Salt and black pepper to taste

4 eggs

Preheat the oven to 375°F. Heat the oil in a large skillet set over medium heat. Add the onion and cook for about 3 minutes until translucent.

Add the mushrooms and cook for about 5 minutes, until lightly browned.

Stir in the bacon, spinach, and chiles and cook for a few minutes, until the spinach is heated through. If any water from the spinach accumulates in the pan, carefully drain. Season with salt and pepper.

Divide the mixture among four 6-ounce oven-safe ramekins that have been lightly greased with butter. Carefully rack an egg into each dish making sure to keep the yolks intact. Place the ramekins in a baking dish and bake until the whites are just set but the yolks are still runny, about 10 minutes. Makes 4 servings.

BLACK BEAN BREAKFAST QUESADILLAS

1 can (24 oz) black beans, rinsed and drained

1 cup shredded reduced-fat Monterey jack cheese

1 jalapeño pepper, thinly sliced

8 small whole wheat tortillas

2 tsp extra-virgin olive oil

1 avocado, pitted, peeled, and sliced

½ lime, cut into wedges.

Preheat the oven to 200°F. Divide the beans, cheese, and pepper evenly among 4 tortillas. Top with the remaining tortillas.

Heat 1 teaspoon of oil in a large nonstick skillet over medium-high heat. Put 2 quesadillas in the pan. Press down with a spatula as they cook.

Shake the pan so they don't stick. Brown for 2 to 4 minutes, flip, and cook the other side until browned and the cheese is melted. Move the finished quesadillas to the oven to keep warm. Then repeat the process with the remaining oil and quesadillas.

Cut the quesadillas into quarters with a pizza cutter or knife. Top each quarter with 2 avocado slices. Squeeze lime juice on top. Makes 4 servings.

FRITTATA WITH ARUGULA & PEPPERS

½ **Tbsp olive oil**

1 **red bell pepper, sliced thinly**

1 **cup sliced mushrooms**

1 **clove garlic**

4 **cups baby arugula or baby spinach**

3 **whole eggs**

3 **egg whites**

Salt and pepper to taste

Herbs and spices to taste

Preheat the broiler. Heat the oil in a nonstick pan over medium heat. Add the sliced bell pepper, mushrooms, and garlic and sauté until softened.

Stir in the arugula and cook for another 2 minutes, until slightly wilted. Meanwhile, whisk together the eggs and egg whites.

Put the eggs on top of the vegetables. Season with salt, pepper, and herbs and spices of your choice. Cook on the stovetop for 5 to 6 minutes, until most of the egg has set.

Place the pan under the broiler and cook for about 3 minutes, until the rest of the egg has fully set and the top begins to brown. Cool slightly, cut into 4 wedges and serve. Makes 2 servings.

Drink This, Lose Weight

Adding a cup (or two) of green tea to your daily diet can help fire your fat furnace in two ways. First, it controls blood sugar and quashes hunger: In a Swedish study that looked at green tea's effect on hunger, researchers divided up participants into two groups: One group sipped water with their meals, and the other group drank green tea. Not only did tea sippers report less of a desire to eat their favorite foods (even two hours after sipping the brew), they found those foods to be less satisfying.

And second, it boosts your calorie burn, especially if you have it before any type of exercise: In a recent 12-week study, participants who combined a daily habit of four to five cups of green tea each day with a 25-minute workout lost an average of two more pounds than the non-tea-drinking exercisers.

It's the power of the unique catechins found in green tea that can blast adipose tissue by triggering the release of fat from fat cells (particularly in the belly), then speeding up the liver's capacity for turning that fat into energy. All this while doing something unique for your heart: A 2015 study from the Institute of Food Research found that the polyphenols in green tea block a "signaling molecule" called VEGF, which in the body can trigger both heart disease and cancer.

DINNER

Working in the restaurant business often means eating at odd hours. When others are sitting down to dinner, you're the one making it. In years past, I would often eat my last meal of the day late into the night, and that habit led to terrible acid reflux and lots of sleepless nights.

I had to learn to listen to my body, and now, I no longer eat past 6 p.m. The practice has cured me of the acid reflux, and I sleep a lot better. Lunch is obviously the biggest meal of the day, when you'll probably have your pizza. So for dinner, you're going to want to keep it light. Here are a few quick and simple recipes to try out.

HOW I LOST 100 POUNDS

For dinner, I'll typically have seafood with a side of beans—protein and fiber. Beans are low on the Glycemic Index, meaning they break down slowly and keep me feeling full longer.

BEEF PATTY WITH GRILLED RED PEPPER

7 oz lean, grass-fed ground beef

Sea salt and cracked black pepper to taste

2 tsp extra-virgin olive oil, divided

1 red bell pepper

Form the beef into a patty and season with salt and pepper.

Heat a stove-top grill pan over medium and cook for about 3 minutes per side for medium-rare.

Remove from the heat and drizzle with 1 teaspoon extra-virgin olive oil.

Slice the pepper in half, removing the seeds and core. Cook in a stove-top grill pan for 5 minutes per side until charred. Drizzle with 1 teaspoon olive oil.

CHICKEN TACOS WITH SALSA VERDE

8 corn tortillas

3 cups shredded rotisserie chicken, skin removed

1½ cups bottled salsa verde

½ cup crumbled Cotija or feta cheese

1 medium onion, minced

1 cup chopped fresh cilantro

2 limes, quartered

Heat the tortillas in a large skillet or sauté pan until lightly toasted.

Combine the chicken with the salsa in a large mixing bowl, then divide evenly among the tortillas.

Top with crumbled cheese, onion, and cilantro.

Serve with lime wedges.

GRILLED CHICKEN WITH GRILLED EGGPLANT

1 8-oz boneless, skinless chicken breast

Sea salt and cracked black pepper to taste

1 eggplant, sliced into ½-inch circles

1 tsp extra-virgin olive oil

2 tsp fresh chopped parsley

Heat a stove-top grill pan over medium heat. Sprinkle the chicken with salt and pepper.

Cook about 5 minutes per side on a grill pan until cooked through.

Place the eggplant slices in the grill pan and cook for 2 minutes on each side until softened. Drizzle with olive oil. Season with salt and parsley.

GRILLED SALMON WITH BAKED BRUSSELS SPROUTS

7 oz Brussels sprouts

2 tsp extra-virgin olive oil, divided

Sea salt and cracked black pepper to taste

1 7-oz salmon fillet

Preheat the oven to 400°F.

Boil the Brussels sprouts for 10 minutes in enough water to cover. Drain and cut each in half.

Transfer to a baking dish and drizzle with 1 teaspoon olive oil. Season with salt and pepper. Bake for 15 minutes.

Heat a stove-top grill pan over medium heat. Season the salmon with salt and pepper. Cook 3 minutes per side for rare, 4 minutes for medium-rare. Remove from the heat and drizzle with 1 teaspoon olive oil.

Serve with a side salad.

GRILLED SHRIMP WITH WHITE BEANS

1 Tbsp extra-virgin olive oil

1 small carrot, diced

1 stalk celery, diced

½ small white onion, diced

1 15-oz canned white beans, drained and rinsed

Sea salt and cracked black pepper to taste

5 fresh or frozen shrimp (defrosted)

Heat 1 tablespoon of extra-virgin olive oil in a pan and sauté the carrot, celery and onion for 5 minutes until softened.

Add to the beans along with ½ cup water. Sprinkle with salt and pepper. Simmer for 10 minutes until the beans begin to break down, most of the liquid evaporates and the consistency becomes like a puree.

Peel and devein the shrimp. Cook in a stove-top grill pan for 2 minutes per side. Plate shrimp atop the bean mixture.

Serve with a side of Greek salad. (Chop 1 tomato, ½ cucumber, and 1 stalk of celery and combine with 2 sliced black olives and 1 teaspoon capers. Dress with 1 teaspoon extra-virgin olive oil.)

GRILLED TURKEY BREAST WITH SPINACH AND AVOCADO SALAD

1 5-oz boneless turkey breast

1 tsp extra-virgin olive oil

1 bunch fresh spinach

½ avocado, chopped

Heat a stove-top grill pan over medium. Cook the turkey breast until cooked through, about 5 minutes per side. Drizzle with 1 teaspoon olive oil.

Wash the spinach and combine with the avocado. Drizzle with Lemon Dressing (recipe on 160)

LEMON DRESSING (FOR SALADS)

¼ cup fresh lemon juice (or balsamic vinegar)

2 tsp Dijon mustard

Sea salt and cracked black pepper to taste

¾ cup extra-virgin olive oil

Add the lemon juice and mustard to a blender and blend with a pinch of salt and pepper.

With the blender running, slowly add the olive oil and blend until the dressing becomes creamy. Store in the refrigerator for up to a week.

THE PIZZA DIET

STEWED BABY OCTOPUS WITH GRILLED VEGETABLES

¼ pound fresh baby octopus, cut into 1-inch pieces

Sea salt and cracked black pepper to taste

2 Tbsp extra-virgin olive oil, divided

1 cup crushed San Marzano tomatoes

2 tsp fresh chopped parsley

1 red bell pepper, sliced into ½-inch strips

1 zucchini, sliced into ½-inch discs

1 eggplant, sliced into ½-inch discs

Clean the octopus and season with salt and pepper. Chop into 1-inch pieces.

Heat 1 tablespoon of extra-virgin olive oil in a sauté pan and add the octopus. Cover and cook for a couple minutes until the octopus goes from gray to red in color.

Add the crushed tomatoes. Remove the lid and simmer for 15 minutes. Add salt and pepper if needed. Sprinkle with chopped parsley before serving.

Heat a stove-top grill pan over medium. Cook the vegetables for 2 minutes on each side. Drizzle with extra-virgin olive oil and sprinkle with salt and pepper.

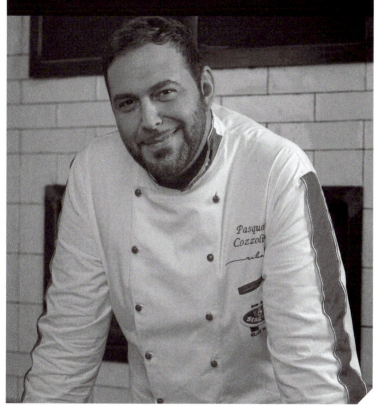

Chapter 9

Can You Really Lose Weight This Deliciously?

Chef Cozzolino answers his fans' most frequently asked questions

C'mon, does this diet really work?

Yes. I am the living proof that eating the Pizza Diet way can help you lose significant weight. But the Pizza Diet does not mean it is okay to eat pizza all the time or as much as you want. The diet works because it is all about eating healthy, whole foods in satisfying but reasonable quantities. Remember that I changed my "American" diet to a more Mediterranean-style diet rich in vegetables, fruits, nuts, whole grains and lean meats and fish. I ate a breakfast that satisfied my hunger but did not cause cravings an hour later. My dinners were low in calories. And I ate a small pizza every day for lunch, made with dough that did not send my blood sugar through the roof. By eliminating that sacrifice part of so many diets that are hard to follow, I made cutting calories and losing weight easy to do. And you can, too.

Will I have trouble following the diet?

It can be difficult to change your lifestyle in the beginning. Stay committed and focused on your goals. And remember, once a week you're treated to a cheat day. That's two or three meals a week in which you can eat pretty much whatever you want. You may indulge in the beginning, but I'll bet as the weeks go by, you'll no longer be tempted by junk food, as your body gets used to eating healthier. Even when you do eat junk, it won't taste as good and you'll no longer crave it.

On a cheat day recently, I sat down to a big bowl of mac and cheese, thinking this was what I wanted. I took one bite and pushed the bowl away. I didn't want it anymore.

How much weight can I expect to lose on the Pizza Diet?

A lot in the first 2 weeks; then your weight will probably plateau. This happens on most diets. Keep at it, and don't become obsessed with the number on the scale. While it's good for your weight to drop, that number can be misleading. What you should really watch is your body fat percentage. Women should aim for between 25 and 31 percent, men 14 to 25 percent. If you're athletic, an even lower percentage.

How can I measure progress?

Step on the scale every 5 days to keep tabs on the big picture. But again, weight is not everything. It's better to measure progress by other terms. Do you have less back pain? Do you have more energy? Are you able to climb stairs without being winded? Has your quality and enjoyment of life increased? Those should be your markers.

Can I alter this diet for my size and weight?

Yes, and you should. These recipes were created for the average person in height and weight. If you find you're not getting results after a few weeks, cut back on the portion sizes.

What if I'm too busy to make a pizza every day?

That's understandable. You may also get tired of eating pizza, believe it or not. Feel free to sub it out with an equally healthy lunch within the same calorie range (550 to 600) or less. Try a

simple whole-wheat pasta (avoid cream sauces) or dishes built
around healthy complex carbs, including legumes, barley, veggies
and nuts.

How long can I stay on this diet?

At least until you reach your goal weight. But remember, it is
a lifestyle, a healthy way of eating you should maintain always.

What if I'm eating out at a restaurant?

It shouldn't be an issue. Make it your cheat day or simply
order a dish that you might find on this plan. Steer clear of anything heavy and fried, and instead opt for grilled proteins, salads
and vegetables.

What if I'm vegetarian?

In this book, you'll find recipes for vegetarians and vegans,
as well.

Can I drink something besides water on this diet?

Definitely. Unsweetened iced tea, black coffee, seltzer. You're
free to have one or two small glasses of beer or wine each day. But
you will lose weight quicker if you avoid all alcoholic beverages.

Should I take any dietary supplements?

Ideally, you should be eating a balanced diet that provides all
the vitamins and minerals your body needs. That said, if you'd
like to add supplements, go right ahead.

Why do people who eat pizza get fat?

It should be pretty clear by now: They're eating the wrong kind of pizza. If you're eating pizza from American chains or from those by-the-slice places, you're essentially eating junk food. I've also found that people who eat fast food–type pizza tend to also eat french fries and ice cream and drink soda. Then they blame the pizza.

HOW I LOST 100 POUNDS

I kept the jeans I could no longer fit into as a motivator to lose my 48-inch "fat pants."

Isn't it important to eat fewer calories in order to lose weight?

Yes, but the point of this diet is to shift the focus away from calories and onto the quality of the food you're eating.

Will yeast make me bloated?

Yeast can lead to bloating and other gastrointestinal ailments. This won't happen with my pizza. The dough is long-leavened, so the yeast disappears.

How can I recognize a good Neapolitan pizza place in the U.S.?

Many restaurants claim to make pizza in the traditional Neapolitan style. They even put the word right on their sign. But chances are, they're not making it the right way.

To see if the pizza you're being served passes the test, first look at the crust. It should be light, not pita-like. It should be puffy around the edges and flat in the middle. When you cut into the crust, you should see large air bubbles.

The website for Associazione Verace Pizza Napoletana, a nonprofit Italian pizza group, contains a list of restaurants in the U.S. that serve real Neapolitan pizza. For the listings, by state, go to americas.pizzanapoletana.org.

Can I use store-bought frozen crust?

It's always preferable to make your own, and most store-bought crusts are loaded with preservatives and other unhealthy ingredients. That said, if you can find a frozen crust with five ingredients or fewer—flour, water, yeast, salt and maybe extra-virgin olive oil—give it a try.

What if I can't find the flour you recommend?

If you cannot find the Italian flour Le 5 Stagioni that I use, you can substitute organic, stone-ground, whole-wheat flour instead. Your pizza will turn out a little different, however. The crust will be darker, the recipe will require more water and the raising time will be less. If you can't find that kind of flour, go for organic 00 flour. But first try looking for Le 5 Stagioni on Amazon.

Why do you only use extra-virgin olive oil?

Quite simply: It's healthy.

Some diets will restrict the quantities of oil you're allowed to consume, but on this diet, I recommend you eat 5 tablespoons of EVOO a day. Use it to cook proteins and drizzle it on your pizzas and salads. Yes, it's high in calories per serving, but just counting calories doesn't make sense. Olive oil contains unsaturated fatty acids essential for metabolic activity and helps our bodies absorb vitamins and nutrients.

EVOO is also more natural and less toxic than other oils. It's made by pressing olives, while most seed oils are extracted via high heat or through the use of chemical solvents.

EVOO also has a relatively high smoke point—the temperature beyond which an oil begins to burn and produce harmful free radicals and potentially cancer-causing compounds. EVOO has a smoke point of 405°F (plain butter is 350°F, by comparison), making it unlikely that you'll burn it while cooking.

Do I really have to eliminate all desserts?

You should try. As I wrote earlier, I recommend you eat no more than 5 teaspoons of sugar a day. The sweetener is toxic, and mounting evidence suggests it may be one of the prime drivers of weight gain. To satisfy your sweet tooth, reach for 50 to 100 grams of dark chocolate a day.

Chapter 10

7-Day Sample Meal Plan

Your Pizza Diet starter menu

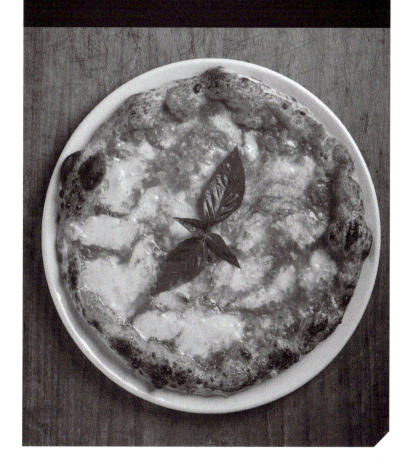

This 1-week plan is taken directly from my own eating program. This is how I ate to lose weight and it's how I eat now to maintain my shape. Give it a try and adapt it to your own preferences. Again, if you find it difficult to eat a pizza during lunchtime, use your pizza as your evening meal, swapping dinner for lunch.

This is simply a guide. Developing your own plan for eating to lose weight is critically important to your ability to stick with it and achieve the results you're looking for.

HOW I LOST 100 POUNDS

I used to deal with stress by snacking. Now I deal with it by kickboxing at the gym.

DAY ONE

Breakfast

½ cup high-fiber, low-sugar cereal or granola with ¼ cup home-made or store-bought, unsweetened almond milk. (Can also use skim milk.) Top with a small handful of raw, sliced almonds.

To make almond milk, combine 2 ounces organic blanched almonds with ⅔ cup warm water in a blender. Blend until smooth. Strain through a cheesecloth into a glass bottle or air-tight container and add a pinch of sea salt. Store in the refrigerator for up to 3 days.

Snack

1 orange

Lunch

Pizza margherita
Side of grilled zucchini

Slice 1 zucchini into ½-inch circles and cook in the grill pan for 2 minutes on each side. Drizzle with a little extra-virgin olive oil and sprinkle with salt and chopped parsley.

Snack

Mix about a half-ounce of granola with 4.5 ounces plain Greek yogurt

Dinner

Grilled Chicken with Grilled Eggplant (156)

DAY TWO

Breakfast
Coffee sweetened with 1 teaspoon pure maple syrup, ½ cup granola and ¼ cup almond milk. Top with fresh strawberries.

Snack
1 orange plus 1 handful of walnuts

Lunch
Marinara pizza
Side salad

Snack
1 Nature Valley Oats 'n Honey granola bar
(They come two to a package.)

Dinner
Grilled Salmon with Baked Brussels Sprouts (157)

DAY THREE

Breakfast

16 ounces fresh-squeezed orange juice

1 apple

1 slice whole-wheat toast, dry

1 sunny-side-up egg

Snack

1 banana

1 small handful of almonds

Lunch

Pizza margherita

Side kale salad: Toss fresh kale with a few cherry tomatoes and raisins. **Top with lemon or balsamic dressing:** Combine ¼ cup fresh lemon juice or balsamic vinegar, 2 teaspoons Dijon mustard and a pinch of sea salt and black pepper in a blender. With the blender running, slowly add ¾ cup extra-virgin olive oil until the dressing becomes creamy. Store in the refrigerator for up to a week.

Snack

1 orange

Dinner

Stewed Baby Octopus with Grilled Vegetables (161)

DAY FOUR

Breakfast
1 cappuccino with skim milk
Bacon, Lettuce, Tomato, and Egg Sandwich (148)

Snack
1 kiwifruit

Lunch
Pizza margherita with grilled vegetables
14 ounces apple juice

Snack
1 pink grapefruit
1 small handful of almonds

Dinner
Beef Patty with Grilled Red Pepper (154)

DAY FIVE

Breakfast
1 cup green or black tea
1 3-inch pancake made from boxed, gluten-free mix, such as Trader Joe's. Top with a drizzle of maple syrup and 1 teaspoon unsalted Irish butter.

Snack
2 slices of fresh pineapple

Lunch
Pizza with broccoli rabe and ground beef
Side salad

Snack
5 ounces fresh cherries
1 small handful of walnuts

Dinner
Grilled Turkey Breast with Spinach and Avocado Salad (159)

DAY SIX

Breakfast
Black Bean Breakfast Quesadilla (150)

Snack
7 ounces fresh cherries

Lunch
Pizza margherita
Side of grilled zucchini

Snack
1 cereal bar
1 orange

Dinner
Grilled Shrimp with White Beans (page 158)

DAY SEVEN (Cheat Day)

Breakfast

1 cup green tea with a splash of almond milk

½ cup cereal with ¼ cup almond milk. Top with raw almonds, walnuts and fresh blueberries. Drizzle with 1 teaspoon maple syrup.

Snack

1 apple

Lunch

Cheat pizza. Feel free to top the base recipe with whatever you'd like, including previously forbidden ingredients such as pepperoni.

Snack

½ can of lentil soup

1 kiwifruit

Dinner

Cheat night. Eat whatever you want.

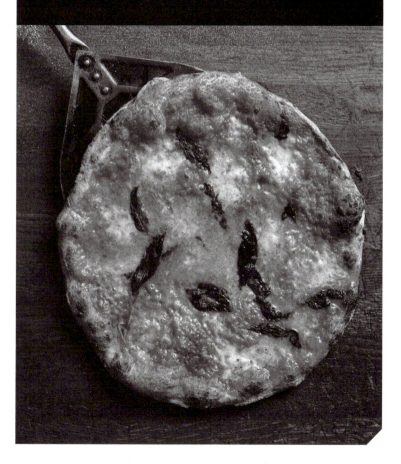

Chapter 11
Avoid a Takeout Pizza Disaster
Worst and best pizzeria pies

181

I recommend that you try to make your own pizzas with my suggested dough most of the time. But I know that sometimes you need to run in to a pizzeria for a slice or you are with friends who are ordering a few pies for a party. In those cases, you help yourself and your health by becoming a mindful eater. In other words, know what you're eating. There are big fat bombs lurking out there in pizzerialand. Most of them can be found in the big pizza chains that try to lure you in with increasingly outrageous pizza gimmicks.

Remember this one? Not long ago, Pizza Hut introduced their artery-clogging, weight-loss-foiling frankenfood, the 15' Hot Dog Bites pie—a large, one-topping pizza with pigs-in-a-blanket baked into the crust!

Unfortunately, Pizza Hut isn't alone in offering pies that better resemble manhole covers than Neapolitan delicacies. At most popular restaurants, thin, healthy crusts have gotten thicker, more bloated with cheap-carb calories. Toppings have gotten gimmicky, so healthy mozzarella and tomato sauces are sometimes replaced with things like burger meat, ziti or chicken fingers. And serving sizes—especially for "individual" pizzas—have taken these pies to a new level of caloric callousness.

It has gotten pretty bad out there. So my friends at *Eat This, Not That!* decided to call out these knucklehead pizzas. The editors researched every pie in America—restaurant and frozen—and determined the absolute worst for your health and waistline. And then they offered a "best list" of pizzas that won't go to your bottom line. Use this as a guide to steering away from the likes of Hot Dog Bites pies and toward healthier options.

CHAIN PIZZERIAS

WORST GIMMICK PIZZA
Pizza Hut Hot Dog Bites Pizza

Estimated per slice: 460 calories, 30 g fat (9.9 g saturated fat), 32.7 g carbohydrates

▶ **That's the fat equivalent of 7.5 Taco Bell Soft Fresco Steak Tacos!**

We've seen Pizza Hut do some kooky things in the past to try to woo new fans—remember the Crazy Cheesy Crust Pizza, with 16 crust pockets of five totally different cheeses? Their latest monster mashup is Hot Dog Bites Pizza—a cheesy, pepperoni pizza surrounded by pigs in a blanket instead of the standard crust. Combining two fattening, calorie-dense, all-American foods is a lose-lose situation (though you won't lose weight)—there's a whopping 3,680 calories in a typical, 8-slice pie, to be exact. Oh, and it's served with French's mustard—for dipping all those hot dogs, of course. Yum?

EAT THIS INSTEAD!
Pizza Hut Skinny Beach Pizza
(1 slice, 14″ large skinny slice)

400 calories, 12 g fat (6 g saturated fat), 880 mg sodium, 56 g carbohydrates

WORST PIZZA SLICE
Sbarro Stuffed Sausage and Pepperoni Pizza (1 slice)

810 calories, 40 g fat (15 g saturated fat), 2,180 mg sodium, 73 g carbohydrates, 36 g protein

▶ **That's the fat equivalent of 10 slices of pan-fried bacon!**

The architecture of this thing makes it less like a slice of pizza and more like a pizza-inspired Chipotle Burrito. It relies on an oversize shell of oily bread to hold together a gooey wad of cheese, sausage and pepperoni. The net result is a pizza pocket with two-thirds of your day's fat and more than a day's worth of sodium. And the traditional pizza slices aren't much better; few fall below 600 calories. If you want to do well at Sbarro, think thin crust with nothing but produce on top.

EAT THIS INSTEAD!
Sbarro New York Style Fresh Tomato Pizza (1 slice)

410 calories, 14 g fat (8 g saturated fat), 790 mg sodium, 53 g carbohydrates, 16 g protein

THE PIZZA DIET

The Scary Chemical Found in Takeout Pizza Boxes

Here's another compelling reason to bake a homemade pizza: Those pizza delivery boxes can last for just about forever, which should raise some eyebrows. Unless you have a ton of extra time on your hands, you probably never wondered why. Sure, cardboard is thicker than your average paper plate, but pizza boxes have also been chemically treated with per-fluoroalkyl substances (PFASs) to withstand the fat dripping from the cheese and meat toppings. While these chemicals help keep your kitchen counter safe from grease, they pose a number of dangers to human health.

In addition to disrupting the immune system, the chemicals may increase the risk of cancer, hypothyroidism, liver malfunction and obesity, according to the U.S. Department of Health and Human Services and international health and environmental experts. Although toxicologists have long been concerned about PFASs, they are just now asking manufacturers to replace the substances with safer alternatives. They also want products laced with the chemicals to be labeled as such to help consumers stay away from the toxins whenever possible.

On the opposing side of the issue, the Environmental Protection Agency says that the chemicals don't pose too much of a threat to our health and are actually safer than alternative options used in the past. Since the verdict is still out, don't expect any major changes to your pizza box any time soon. In the mean time, if PFASs concern you, minimize your exposure by taking your favorite pizza delivery place off speed dial and eating at the restaurant or making your own pizza at home.

WORST PIZZA WANNABE
Romano's Macaroni Grill Smashed Meatball Fatbread

1,420 calories, 59 g fat (28 g saturated fat), 2,970 mg sodium, 149 g carbohydrates

▶ **That's the calorie equivalent of almost 17 Eggo Confetti Waffles!**

That is not a typo: Romano's loudly advertises their "fatbread"—baked dough smothered with cheese and toppings—as being "fat on crust, fat on toppings and fat on flavor" but they should have added "fat on you." Consuming more than half of your daily calories in one sitting is just asking for a 3 p.m. desktop snooze and a fatter tummy. Skip them and choose a simpler pasta instead. (But beware: Ravioli alla Vodka and the Penne Arrabbiata are 2 of only 4 lunchtime pastas with fewer than 1,000 calories.)

EAT THIS INSTEAD!
Ravioli à la Vodka

660 calories, 37 g fat, (20 g saturated fat), 1,440 mg sodium, 50 g carbohydrates

WORST PIZZA FOR KIDS
CiCi's Pizza Buffet Mac & Cheese
(two 12″ Buffet Pizza Slices)

380 calories, 9 g fat (4 g saturated fat), 880 mg sodium, 60 g carbohydrates

▶ **That's the carb equivalent of shotgunning more than 4 slices of Wonder Bread!**

Macaroni and cheese pizza? While it might seem like the best idea ever to kids the world over, this cute concept is potentially disastrous for your health—and your children's. Why top an already carbohydrate-heavy dish with more carbs, not to mention fat? While the calorie count doesn't register as high as most problematic pies on this list, that's only because the slices are tiny; believe us, in CiCi's all-you-can-eat environment, the damage can add up quickly. But if you bring one of their pizzas home, celebrate their smaller slices as built-in portion control—and go with flatbread. The kids will love the crunch.

EAT THIS INSTEAD!
Cheese Flatbread (2 slices)

200 calories, 9 g fat (5 g saturated fat), 380 mg sodium, 24 g carbohydrates

WORST SEAFOOD PIZZA
Red Lobster Lobster Pizza

680 calories, 31 g fat (12 g saturated fat), 1,740 mg sodium, 66 g carbohydrates

▶ **That's the fat equivalent of 442 large shrimp! Really.**

Fare from the sea is typically a healthy way to go, but sprinkle it over a bed of starchy dough and fatty cheese and you have a different story altogether. Billed as a starter, this Lobster Pizza is the only pizza on Red Lobster's menu—luckily it shares space with one of the world's greatest appetizers: shrimp cocktail.

EAT THIS INSTEAD!
Chilled Jumbo Shrimp Cocktail

120 calories, 1 g fat, 590 mg sodium, 9 g carbohydrates

WORST MASHUP PIZZA
Papa John's Fritos Chili Pizza (2 slices)
720 calories, 30 g fat (12 g saturated fat), 1,400 mg sodium

▶ **That's the sodium equivalent of dumping 5 salt packets into your mouth!**

Papa John's seasonal concoction of pizza, beef chili and yes, Fritos is an insult to almost every cuisine known to man. By our estimates, a whole pie would come salted up with nearly 6,000 mg of sodium! A better defense is a good offense, so start your meal off here with a few pieces of belly-filling protein in the form of wings or chicken strips. Consider it insurance against scarfing too many slices later on.

EAT THIS INSTEAD!
The Works Original Crust Pizza
(1 slice, large pie) and Chickenstrips (3) with Cheese Dipping Sauce
400 calories, 26 g fat (8.5 g saturated fat), 1,060 mg sodium

WORST PIZZA IN AMERICA
Uno Chicago Grill Chicago Classic Deep Dish Individual Pizza

2,300 calories, 164 g fat (53 g saturated fat, 1 g trans fat), 4,910 mg sodium, 119 g carbohydrates

▶ **That's the sodium equivalent of 27 small bags of Lay's Potato Chips!**

The problem with deep-dish pizza (which Uno's knows a thing or two about since they invented it back in 1943) is not just the extra empty calories and carbs from the crust, it's that the thick, doughy base provides the structural integrity to house extra heaps of cheese, sauce, and greasy toppings. The result is an individual pizza with more calories than you should eat in a day. Oh, did we mention it has nearly 3 days' worth of saturated fat, too? The key to (relative) success at Uno's lies in their flatbread pies—and share them!

EAT THIS INSTEAD!
Cheese and Tomato Flatbread Pizza (½ pizza)

490 calories, 23.5 g fat (11 g saturated fat), 1,290 mg sodium, 48 g carbohydrates

11 BELLY-TIGHTENING TIPS FOR PIZZA DIET SUCCESS
Easy Extra Efforts Can Speed the Results of Your Weight Loss

1. Eat Mushrooms, Drop Pounds

If you substituted portobello or white button mushrooms for beef just once a week, you'd save more than 20,000 calories and roughly 1,500 grams of fat (and shed more than five pounds!) over the course of a year without changing anything else about your diet. Researchers at Johns Hopkins Weight Management Center found that choosing low-energy-density foods, specifically white button mushrooms, instead of high-energy-density foods such as ground beef, can help prevent obesity. For four days, their study subjects saved 420 calories and 30 grams of fat per day by eating mushroom lasagna, napoleons, sloppy joes, and vegetable chili entrees. "The best thing about using mushrooms as a dietary substitute is that you typically won't compensate for the lower-calorie meal by eating more food later in the day," says study author Lawrence Cheskin, MD, director of Johns Hopkins Weight Management Center.

2. Decorate Your Plate

A 14-year study found that men whose diets were highest in colorful fruits and vegetables had a 70 percent lower risk of digestive-tract cancers. How to reach your quota: Never eat a meal that doesn't contain a vegetable or fruit. And no, fries don't count. The color of produce can tip you off to its nutritional value:

Below are five color categories of fruits and vegetables and their known health benefits. Get at least five servings a day. (One serving equals 1 cup raw or ½ cup cooked.)

Blues and Purples: Blueberries, blackberries, purple grapes, plums, raisins, eggplant. *Benefits:* Keep memory sharp and reduce risk of many types of cancer, including prostate cancer

Greens: Kiwi, honeydew, spinach, broccoli, romaine lettuce, Brussels sprouts, cabbage. *Benefits:* Protect bones, teeth, and eyesight

Whites: Pears, bananas, mushrooms, cauliflower, onions, garlic. *Benefits:* Lower LDL cholesterol and reduce risk of heart disease

Yellows and Oranges: Oranges, grapefruit, peaches, cantaloupe, mangoes, pineapple, squash, carrots. *Benefits:* Boost immune system and help prevent eye disease

Reds: Watermelon, strawberries, raspberries, cranberries, cherries, tomatoes, radishes, red apples. *Benefits:* Help prevent Alzheimer's disease and improve blood flow to the heart

3. End Your Workout with a PB&J

According to nutrition scientists at McMaster University in Hamilton, Ontario, the perfect post-weight-training meal contains 20 to 30 grams of protein (to build new muscle) and 50 to 65 grams of carbohydrates (to repair muscle) and about 400 calories. A peanut butter and jelly sandwich hits that formula deliciously.

4. Extinguish Overeating

Have trouble cutting yourself off after you've eaten your fill? Light a candle when you sit down to the dinner table and blow it out after you've finished your meal. This simple action sends a message to your brain—and your mouth—that it's time to stop noshing. Not only will this strategy keep the temporary food baby that develops when you overeat at bay, over time, eating fewer calories adds up to major weight loss.

5. Eat Oats for Energy

Eat a power breakfast of steel-cut oats topped with chopped walnuts, raisins, and flaxseeds and low-fat milk. The long-burning carbs and protein will fuel your body and brain for hours. Wash it down with orange juice. A University of Alabama study found that getting 400 mg of vitamin C per day significantly reduces the secretion of energy-draining stress hormones.

6. Put a Fork in It

Eat slower and you'll likely eat less because you'll give your belly time to signal your brain that you are full. Do it by holding your fork in your nondominant hand. Bring plenty of napkins.

7. Save 400 Calories with This Dessert

Love your apple pie à la mode? Try this instead: chop up a large crisp apple, dump in in a bowl and top it with 1 cup of plain yogurt (Greek or regular). Sprinkle cinnamon on top. You'll save yourself at least 400 calories and get a healthy dose of protein by avoiding that ice-cream-covered sugar bomb.

8. Eat Cottage Cheese Before Bed

For some people, completely avoiding food before bedtime can actually be bad for their weight-loss goals. First, going to bed with a rumbling tummy makes falling asleep difficult. Second, people who wake up feeling hungry are far more likely to pig out on a big breakfast. Have a little cottage cheese before bed. Not only is it rich in casein protein, it also contains the amino acid tryptophan.

9. Don't Forget Your Lunch

Thinking about what you ate for lunch could keep you from bingeing on afternoon snacks. In a study, subjects were told they were taste-testing three different types of salted popcorn. They were encouraged to eat as much as they wanted. Interestingly, those who were first asked to recall exactly what they had eaten for lunch consumed 30 percent less popcorn than those who didn't review their lunch menu beforehand. The researchers say that taking a few seconds to remember what you had during a recent meal might enhance awareness of how satiating the food was, which then might reduce future noshing.

10. Chew More, Weigh Less

Replace a glass of apple juice with a whole apple. A study in the *International Journal of Obesity* reports that people reduced their daily calorie intake by up to 20 percent when they substituted a piece of fruit for fruit juice with their lunch. The researchers say that chewing stimulates satiety hormones, and whole food takes longer for your intestines to process, helping you to feel fuller longer and consume less.

11. Go Heavy on the Vinegar

Enjoy that submarine sandwich, even with all that Italian bread, by adding extra vinegar. The acetic acid in the vinegar interferes with enzymes that break down carbohydrates, keeping blood sugar levels from rising quickly, say nutritionists at Arizona State University. You can also get the same result by starting a high-carb meal with a salad drizzled with vinaigrette.

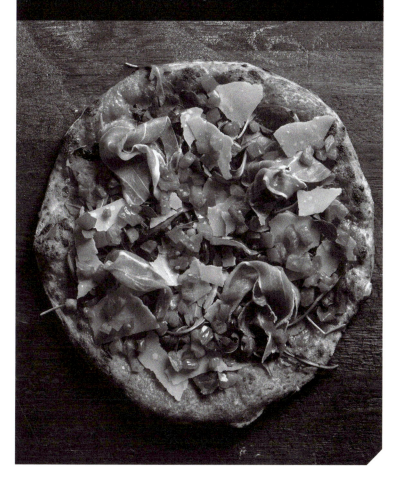

Chapter 12

Life after the Pizza Diet
(more pizza!)

By now, you should have all the knowledge and materials you need to embark on this journey. You should be ready to start changing your life, eating differently and confusing your friends by telling them you're on something called the "pizza diet." Don't worry about it. I still get a few raised eyebrows.

What your bewildered friends may not understand is that this isn't really a diet at all. It's a lifestyle. You're going from eating in the unhealthy, American-style way to the healthier Mediterranean way. And well-made pizza just happens to be part of that.

This is about thinking differently about the kinds of food you eat and redefining the relationship between food and your body. Don't think about this new lifestyle as depriving yourself of anything. You're not making any sacrifices. You get to eat a delicious pizza every single day. Keep that at the forefront of your brain.

As for that other stuff you'll no longer be eating, it's important not to focus on what you're missing. Instead, focus on what you could be gaining. Don't think, "I wish I could have that bag of cookies." Think, "Isn't it great that I left my old life behind and I'm no longer someone who eats an entire box of Nilla Wafers?"

Remember why you decided to buy this book and start making changes in the first place. Never forget that.

As I mentioned in a previous chapter, I kept the size-42 pants I was hoping to fit into out in plain view so I could see them every day and refocus on my goal. I also like to post that week's meal plan on the refrigerator as another visual reminder.

Find something for yourself and use it to provide motivation.

It's also important that you don't become too militant. Don't beat yourself up if you're out at a restaurant and eat something you shouldn't or if your weight loss trails off. I was recently in Italy for a week to judge the world pizza championships. While I was there, I ate much more than I normally do (how could I not?) and gained a couple pounds. But once I got back to New York, I fell right back into the diet and didn't stray.

After a few months, you can also start swapping out foods on the plan. If you get tired of pizza—something that strangely never happens to me—have something else for lunch instead, such as a whole-wheat pasta. As long as it's sensible, isn't loaded with cream and has around 600 calories or less, as the pizza does, go for it.

Some other tips moving forward:

Eat vegetables as an appetizer

Skip the pasta and bread, and instead start your meal with a salad or a serving of boiled vegetables. It could help you eat less of the main course, and the fiber from the vegetables may help you process your meal more effectively and slow the absorption of sugars. (The same advice applies on cheat days for when you're planning on downing a piece of cake or a doughnut. Preface the snack with a helping of vegetables to keep your body from absorbing all the sugar.)

Fight constipation

Starting a new diet can sometimes lead to things getting backed up. To get things moving, add more green, leafy vegetables, bran, yogurt or almond milk to your meal plan.

Eat on smaller dishes

Research has shown that food served on a smaller plate proved more satisfying than the same amount served on a larger one. The strategy tricks the brain into thinking we're eating more food than we actually are. One Georgia Institute of Technology study discovered that shifting from a 12-inch plate to a 10-incher resulted in a 22 percent decrease in calories consumed at a meal.

Start chewing better

There's a correlation between thinness and the tendency to chew food slowly and thoroughly. Research has shown that the longer you chew each bite, the slower you eat. And the slower you eat, the less you tend to eat.

Chewing food thoroughly also increases the amount of nutrition your body is able to take from food.

Eat candy (but only this one time)

If you're coming to a meal with a particularly robust appetite, munch on a small piece of candy first. The sugar in the candy will immediately raise your blood sugar level, help reduce your appetite and keep you from gorging.

Dine more frequently

Instead of three meals a day, you may want to try eating five or six smaller meals. The plan helps promote an active metabolism, keeps your insulin from spiking, and prevents your digestive system from getting overloaded.

Don't skip meals

Going a few hours without food will force your body to switch into safety mode and begin storing fat. If you're coming off a particularly large lunch, for example, don't opt out of dinner. Instead, eat as you normally would, perhaps opting for a heavier portion of vegetables.

Eat unrefined grains to improve your skin

Got dry skin, acne or eczema? You might want to up your consumption of whole, unrefined grains, such as brown rice and potatoes. Highly refined grains and sugar can lead to inflammation, worsening skin issues.

Eat more lemons

They may help with joint pain and improve the cardiovascular system. You can always swap out the vinegar in a salad dressing for fresh lemon juice, for example.

Keep working out

Once you see your body changing, it won't be hard to stay motivated. And by all means, don't obsess over your weight. I recommend you weigh yourself every five days, not every day, so you don't become fixated on the daily ups and downs and you can get a clearer picture of your long-term progress.

You probably got into this for reasons beyond a number on a scale anyway. You probably want to feel better about yourself, become healthier and reclaim your old body. Who would have thought pizza might be part of the solution?

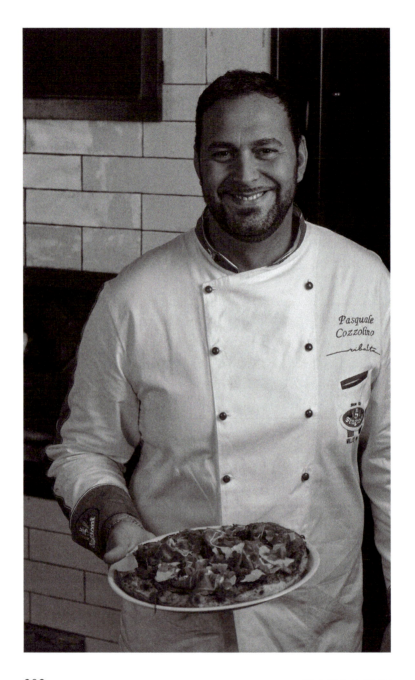

Acknowledgments

Writing a book is an exciting and challenging task, especially when it is your first book. When you are writing that book in English, not in your native language of Italian, the task is so much more difficult, at times frustrating, and slow. Fortunately, I had the help of many patient people. Without them, I would not have found my voice in this new language and never would have been able to complete the book without becoming crazy!

I have many people to thank, beginning with my parents, Rita and Francesco, who encouraged me when I was young and lazy and who spent many hours discussing ideas for the book with me. My wife, Jordie, was starting a new job at the same time I was writing. Thank you, Jordie, for your sacrifice as I wrote every day and for your advice on its creation. I love you. To my sons, Francesco and Lorenzo, I want you to know that your smiles and laughs were a great morale booster as I worked. And you both inspired me to change my lifestyle to lose weight and become healthier physically and psychologically.

I am very grateful to Claudine Ko, a writer for the *New York Post*, who first told the Pizza Diet story in the newspaper, to Haleil Ebe, Miss Mangiapia, who believed in me, and Kekko of the band Modà for the soundtrack I used during my exercise for motivation.

Thank you to Italian nutrition expert Giovanni Moscarella for his amazing advice to me about my diet. Giovanni, you are like a little bird who taught a plane to fly. And to Rosario Procino, my partner in Ribalta restaurants in New York City and Atlanta, for your generous support and friendship throughout this project.

Many thanks to David Zinczenko and the team at Galvanized Media, specifically Michael Freidson, George Karabotsos, and my editor Jeff Csatari, for giving me the opportunity to write this book and guiding me through the process with patience and professionalism. Thanks also to Random House, photographer Jennifer May, writer Reed Tucker who presented my words and recipes in English and Hall Powell, who corrected the scientific and historical material in the book, and encouraged me to press on when I wished to be anywhere but in front of my computer. Thank you to all of my friends who believed in me even when I was discouraged; we will have a toast at the bar.

And, finally, a message to the readers of *The Pizza Diet*: If you are insecure about your body and your weight, I know how you feel. Do not be discouraged. I know that you will succeed and you will feel happy again if you learn to eat healthy foods without sacrificing the foods you love. A big hug and a kiss to you: everything is possible if you really want it.

—*Pizza Maker and Chef Pasquale Cozzolino*

Appendix
GUIDE TO THE BEST
AND WORST FROZEN PIZZA

A ccording to the USDA, when your pizza resembles the right mix of food groups, that pie–even frozen pizza–can provide you with 37 percent of your bone-building calcium, 30 percent of your satiating fiber, 35 percent of your muscle-replenishing protein, and over 50 percent of your recommended intake of lycopene (an antioxidant found in tomatoes that may possess anti-cancer benefits). The trouble in the frozen food aisle is that many frozen pizza options are loaded with preservatives and artery-clogging trans fats. *Eat This, Not That!* looked behind the frosted glass in the supermarket and identified the best and worst frozen pizzas.

TRADITIONAL CHEESE PIZZA

EAT THIS!
AMY'S CHEESE

Nutrition (⅓ pizza, 123 g): 290 calories, 12 g fat (5 g saturated fat), 590 mg sodium, 33 g carbs (2 g fiber, 4 g sugar), 12 g protein

Amy's pizza is made with organic tomatoes, which is important as scientists have found this pesticide-free version of the red fruit actually has higher levels of cancer-fighting lycopene. Bonus: There's no refined wheat or sugar, which means this pie offers more nutritional bang for your buck.

NOT THAT!
RED BARON CLASSIC CRUST
4 CHEESE, 2 PEPPERONI

Nutrition (¼ pizza, 149 g): 390 calories, 17 g fat (9 g saturated fat), 750 mg sodium, 42 g carbs (2 g fiber, 8 g sugar), 16 g protein

If we were to ask you to guess the ingredients in pizza, you'd probably say cheese, tomatoes, and a wheat-yeast crust. We'd bet you wouldn't guess "L-Cysteine hydrochloride" (a salt used to treat overdoses) and "ammonium sulfate" (a commonly-used lawn fertilizer), which are two ingredients found in this franken-pizza. Oh, and did we mention the calorie, fat, and sodium contents are some of the highest on the market?

EAT THIS!
TRADER JOE'S WOOD FIRED UNCURED PEPPERONI PIZZA

Nutrition (⅓ pizza, 144 g): 390 calories, 19 g fat (7 g saturated fat), 840 mg sodium, 40 g carbs (3 g fiber, 4 g sugar), 16 g protein

When nabbing a good ol' pepperoni pizza, we'd recommend a pie that uses uncured pepperoni. Uncured just means the meat is free from chemical nitrates, which have been known to form carcinogenic compounds under conditions of high heat (like, say, a 400-degree oven).

NOT THAT!
TOMBSTONE ORIGINAL PEPPERONI

Nutrition (¼ pizza, 153 g): 390 calories, 20 g fat (8 g saturated fat), 880 mg sodium, 37 g carbs (4 g fiber, 6 g sugar), 18 g protein

Along with containing two, pesticide-ridden, genetically modified oils (corn and soybean), this pizza adds nitrates and other dangerous preservatives to their pepperoni, namely BHA and BHT. Butylated hydroxytoluene (BHT) and Butylated hydroxyanisole (BHA) are both already banned in the UK, Australia, New Zealand, Japan, and much of Europe because they are thought to be carcinogenic.

THIN CRUST

EAT THIS!
NEWMAN'S OWN THIN & CRISPY PEPPERONI

Nutrition (⅓ pie, 125 g): 320 calories, 16 g fat (6 g saturated fat), 800 mg sodium, 31 g carbs (2 g fiber), 15 g protein

Newman's also skips out on the pepperoni laced with nitrates—which, besides serving as a precursor for carcinogenic compounds, also may interfere with the body's natural ability to process sugar and increase the risk for diabetes. Those who have had the pleasure of tasting this "better than takeout" pizza love that the crust is crispy and thin without tasting crackery and is full of grains and flaxseed.

NOT THAT!
RED BARON THIN & CRISPY PEPPERONI PIZZA

Nutrition (⅓ pie, 149 g): 390 calories, 19 g fat (9 g saturated fat), 1,010 mg sodium, 41 g carbs (2 g fiber, 9 g sugar), 14 g protein

Even the Baron's thin-crust pies pack too much of all the bad stuff, including fat, saturated fat, sodium, and MSG in disguise—hydrolyzed soy protein. This appetitive-revving additive may interfere with your hunger hormones, causing you to eat beyond your fill.

VEGGIE

EAT THIS!
NEWMAN'S OWN THIN & CRISPY ROASTED VEGETABLE

Nutrition (⅓ pizza, 135 g): 240 calories, 9 g fat (3.5 g saturated fat), 550 mg sodium, 33 g carbs (3 g fiber, 3 g sugar), 11 g protein

A fire-roasted trio of bell peppers, mushrooms, and red onions top this multigrain thin and crispy crust pizza. It's also higher in fiber and lower in sugar than its alternative.

NOT THAT!
BON APPETIT ROASTED VEGETABLE

Nutrition (⅓ pizza, 136 g): 300 calories, 13 g fat (7 g saturated fat), 430 mg sodium, 35 g carbs (2 g fiber, 8 g sugar), 12 g protein

It might have the same veggies, but where Bon Appetit goes awry is in the additives, using vegetable oils, MSG derivatives, and preservatives. All three have been known to contribute to chronic inflammation, a common culprit of weight gain.

RISING CRUST

EAT THIS!
DIGIORNO ITALIAN SAUSAGE

Nutrition (⅙ pizza, 143 g): 330 calories, 14 g fat (6 g saturated fat), 760 mg sodium, 37 g carbs (1 g fiber, 5 g sugar), 15 g protein

We don't typically recommend grabbing a slice with an equivalent amount of calories as a personal pie, but in this category, we'd rather you go with DiGiorno than the alternatives. This pie has better nutritionals and better ingredients than the one listed below. (And we hear it tastes pretty good, too.)

NOT THAT!
FRESCHETTA OLD FASHIONED SAUSAGE

Nutrition (⅙ pizza, 134 g): 340 calories, 13 g fat (6 g saturated fat), 840 mg sodium, 40 g carbs (2 g fiber, 8 g sugar), 14 g protein

Though similar in calories, this pizza still manages to pack in more sodium, carbs, and sugar than the Eat This option. Even worse is the inclusion of hydrogenated soybean oil, which isn't as dangerous as partially hydrogenated, but may still contain remnants of artery-clogging trans fats from the chemical process used to make it. Don't worry, not all fats are bad.

GLUTEN FREE

EAT THIS! (IT'S A TIE!)
SMART FLOUR CLASSIC CHEESE

Nutrition (½ pizza, 143 g): 350 calories, 14 g fat (7 g saturated fat), 850 mg sodium, 43 g carbs (3 g fiber, 5 g sugar), 13 g protein

This thin-crusted pie is the real deal; you won't even realize it's gluten free! Smart Flour has their own proprietary blend of nutrient-dense ancient grains, including sorghum, teff, and amaranth. They were a little heavy-handed on the sodium, though, so be sure to drink water while you're eating a slice.

UDI'S GF THREE CHEESE PIZZA

Nutrition (½ pizza, 142 g): 360 calories, 15 g fat (9 g saturated fat), 570 mg sodium, 45 g carbs (2 g fiber, 6 g sugar), 12 g protein

Udi's pie has similar nutritionals to Smart Flour, but it's lower in sodium. Pick up this GF standard, made with brown rice flour, and a blend of mozzarella, fontina, and romano cheeses.

NOT THAT!
GLUTINO GF DUO CHEESE

Nutrition (1 pizza, 175 g): 410 calories, 19 g fat (8 g saturated fat), 660 mg sodium, 48 g carbs (3 g fiber, 4 g sugar), 12 g protein

Don't be a glutton with this personal pizza. Glutino's pies are consistently high in calories and fat—and a Not That!

PERSONAL

EAT THIS!
AMY'S LIGHT & LEAN CHEESE PIZZA

Nutrition (1 pizza, 142 g): 270 calories, 6 g fat (3 g saturated fat), 480 mg sodium, 38 g carbs (3 g fiber, 6 g sugar), 14 g protein

One of the best frozen pies on the market, Amy's lightens up a classic pizza by using a low-fat mozzarella but still keeps all the flavor you know and love.

NOT THAT!
DIGIORNO SMALL-SIZE, FOUR-CHEESE TRADITIONAL

Nutrition (1 pizza, 260 g): 710 calories, 29 g fat (14 g saturated fat), 1,190 mg sodium, 88 g carbs (4 g fiber, 12 g sugar), 25 g protein

If you're going to market a pizza as being "personal size," you can't fault us for providing nutritional information for the whole pie—even though DiGiorno deceptively calls the serving size half a pie.

PESTO

EAT THIS!
AMY'S PESTO PIZZA

Nutrition (⅓ pizza, 128 g): 310 calories, 12 g fat (3.5 g saturated fat), 480 mg sodium, 39 g carbs (2 g fiber, 3 g sugar), 12 g protein
Organic basil and pine nuts make up the traditional pesto that flavors up this pie.

NOT THAT!
BON APPETIT MOZZARELLA & PESTO

Nutrition (⅓ pizza, 125 g): 310 calories, 14 g fat (7 g saturated fat), 410 mg sodium, 34 g carbs (2 g fiber, 8 g sugar), 12 g protein
Don't be fooled into thinking this pie is healthy because the brand's name is wishing you good eating. Bon Appetit's pizza may look similar in nutritionals to Amy's at first glance, but there's no reason this pie should have 5 more grams of sugar. There's also no need to compile a list of 37 ingredients, many of which are artificial flavors, preservatives, and trans fats in disguise (mono and diglycerides and hydrogenated cottonseed oil).

CHEESE BLEND

EAT THIS!
AMERICAN FLATBREAD TOMATO SAUCE & THREE CHEESE

Nutrition (½ pizza, 128 g): 300 calories, 10 g fat (5 g saturated fat), 700 mg sodium, 37 g carbs (2 g fiber, 1 g sugar), 15 g protein

If you want a farm-fresh pie without stepping in manure, pick up this pie in the frozen food section. American Flatbread uses mostly organic ingredients and sources cheese from Vermont that is made with milk from Jersey cows.

NOT THAT!
DIGIORNO PIZZERIA! FOUR CHEESE

Nutrition (¼ pizza, 130 g): 310 calories, 13 g fat (6 g saturated fat), 700 mg sodium, 35 g carbs (2 g fiber, 3 g sugar), 12 g protein

Another DiGiorno don't. And in this case, more cheese means more sodium and fat, with none of the extra protein.

CHICKEN

EAT THIS!
NEWMAN'S OWN THIN & CRISPY BBQ RECIPE CHICKEN

Nutrition (⅓ pizza, 133 g): 290 calories, 9 g fat (5 g saturated fat), 750 mg sodium, 36 g carbs (2 g fiber, 6 g sugar), 17 g protein

Newman's Own uses real diced white chicken meat (instead of the rib meat you'll find in CPK's version). They also use an actual barbecue sauce rather than a mixture of molasses and food dye.

NOT THAT!
CALIFORNIA PIZZA KITCHEN CRISPY THIN CRUST BBQ CHICKEN

Nutrition (⅓ pizza, 139 g): 300 calories, 11 g fat (5 g saturated fat), 640 mg sodium, 35 g carbs (1 g fiber, 8 g sugar), 16 g protein

California Pizza Kitchen somehow managed to compile the longest ingredient list of all the frozen pizzas on the market. Among the 50+ items is caramel color, an ingredient known to be contaminated by carcinogens.

MINI PIZZA BAGELS

EAT THIS!
ANNIE'S MINI PIZZA BAGELS UNCURED PEPPERONI

Nutrition (4 pieces, 84 g): 200 calories, 6 g fat (2.5 g saturated fat), 500 mg sodium, 27 g carbs (2 g fiber, 3 g sugar), 10 g protein

Pepperoni pizza bagels are genius; they combine three culinary favorites that are often considered to be diet no-no's to create a tasty snack that's fairly easy on the waistline. They're even more so when they're made without nitrates like in this version. Kids and adults alike are sure to love their compact, portion-controlled size and big flavor.

NOT THAT!
BAGEL BITES CHEESE & PEPPERONI

Nutrition (4 bites, 88 g): 200 calories, 6 g fat (2.5 g saturated fat), 340 mg sodium, 28 g carbs (2 g fiber, 3 g sugar), 7 g protein

They may be the original, but now that there's a better option with cleaner ingredients, you can leave Bagel Bites in the past.

SUPREME

EAT THIS!
NEWMAN'S OWN THIN & CRISPY SUPREME

Nutrition (⅓ pie, 139 g): 320 calories, 15 g fat (5 g saturated fat), 750 mg sodium, 33 g carbs (3 g fiber, 3 g sugar), 14 g protein

When going deluxe, you have to be willing to sacrifice something if you want to stick to your body goals. Luckily, this pie subs out an unnecessary carb-laden crust for a crispy base, allowing you to indulge in the extra meat and veggies, guilt free.

NOT THAT!
RED BARON CLASSIC CRUST SPECIAL DELUXE

Nutrition (⅕ pizza, 130 g): 310 calories, 14 g fat (6 g saturated fat), 670 mg sodium, 34 g carbs (2 g fiber, 7 g sugar), 12 g protein

Even though the nutritional counts aren't dramatically different between this slice and the Eat This! recommendation, this Red Baron option is actually only about a fifth of the pie (and 130 g) as opposed to a third (and 139 g). And like many of its siblings, this guy's also loaded with extra ingredients and preservatives that aren't necessary.

Recipe Index

THE PIZZA DIET

ABOUT THE AUTHOR

Pasquale Cozzolino is the executive chef and co-owner of Ribalta restaurants (ribaltapizzarestaurant.com) in Manhattan and Atlanta.

Born in Naples, Italy, he attended six years of culinary school, where he learned 200-year-old recipes and perfected the art of making Neapolitan Pizza Margherita. After graduation, Pasquale worked for 10 years as a private executive chef in concert tours throughout Europe and South America serving such bands as U2, Madonna, Muse, and Coldplay. In 2011, he moved to New York City to pursue his dream of becoming a pizza chef and owning a restaurant.

In the U.S., Pasquale packed on the pounds by eating American-style fast food. He became dangerously overweight and realized he had to change his lifestyle or risk a heart attack. The answer was pizza, but not just any pizza. Pasquale used top-quality ingredients and his talent for mixing tradition with innovation to develop healthy recipes for pizza so he could lose weight and transform his health while still enjoying Neapolitan cuisine. His creations earned Ribalta New York magazine's best pizza of NYC award.

While eating this pizza every day for lunch, Pasquale lost more than 100 pounds in 7 months—and *The Pizza Diet* was born. Now leaner, healthier, and happier, Pasquale is eager to share his strategies and recipes to help others achieve a healthier lifestyle.

Pasquale lives in Queens, NY, with his wife and two sons.